JUDITH WILLS

COMPLETE SPEED SLIMMING SYSTEM

KT-432-893

Also by Judith Wills
SIZE 12 IN 21 DAYS

JUDITH WILLS

COMPLETE SPEED SLIMMING SYSTEM

YOUR ULTIMATE GUIDE TO QUICKEST-EVER FAT LOSS AND FIGURE RESHAPING

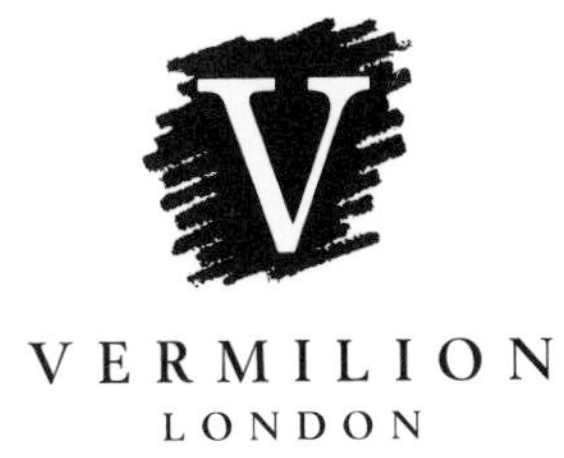

VERMILION
LONDON

WARNING

If you have a medical condition, or are pregnant, the diets and exercises described in this book should not be followed without first consulting your doctor. All guidelines and warnings should be read carefully and the author and publisher cannot accept responsibility for injuries or damage arising out of a failure to comply with the same.

First published 1993 by Vermilion
an imprint of Ebury Press
Random House UK Ltd
Random House
20 Vauxhall Bridge Road
LONDON SW1V 2SA

Text copyright © Judith Wills 1993
Photographs pages 73–89 and 103–117 © Jon Stewart 1993
Photographs pages 91–102 © Tony Allen 1993
Designed by Roger Walker

The right of Judith Wills to be identified as the author of this book has been asserted by her in accordance with the Copyright, Designs and Patents Act, 1988.

All rights reserved. No part of this publication may be reproduced, stored in a retrieval system, or transmitted in any form or by any means, electronic, mechanical, photocopying, recording or otherwise, without the prior permission of the copyright owner.

A catalogue record for this book is available from the British Library

ISBN 0 09 177447 0

Printed in England by Clays Ltd, St Ives plc

CREDITS:
Leotards and leggings courtesy of Dance Bizarre.
Step XT and hand weights courtesy of Espree Fitness Equipment Ltd.
Black trainers available at Olympus Sport, 301 Oxford Street, London W1

CONTENTS

Introduction: Now Everyone Can Lose Weight Quickly! 7

1 Speed Slimming: How It Will Work For You 9

2 Fast Weight Loss: All Your Questions Answered 13

3 How Much Weight Do You Need To Lose? 18

4 The Speed Slimming Diet Programme 25

5 The Sliding-Scale Diets 30

6 The Speed-Plus Plan 55

7 Speed Slimming Recipes 57

8 The Fat Burning Routine 70

9 The Body Shaping Routine 84

10 Staying Slim 118

Food Charts 126

Index of Recipes 144

Introduction: Now Everyone Can Lose Weight Quickly!

How would you like to lose weight fast – and keep it off? For anyone who does want to get slim quickly ... but doesn't want to follow a crash or fad diet; for anyone who wants to see weight coming off at more than just a pound or so a week but who still wants to eat real, tasty, satisfying, filling meals – the Complete Speed Slimming System is the answer.

Whether you need to lose several stone, one stone or just half a stone, you'll find that the weight comes off, week after week, or day after day, right down to target! And at the same time you can be absolutely certain that you're not damaging your health in any way. The methods in this book are tried and tested, and all the diet and exercise advice is safe and sensible.

The Complete Speed Slimming System works to help you shed weight quickly and consistently for the following reasons:

- It increases your metabolic rate (the rate at which your body burns fat and calories) through a unique high-carbohydrate, low-fat dieting system and activity programme.
- It burns off fat, without pain or strain, through the right kind of exercise – a low-intensity programme that is suitable for everyone.
- It tailors the diet and exercise programme to suit you, with the help of special diet, metabolism, shape and fitness questionnaires. No hunger, no deprivation and no misery; for once, you're on the system that's right for you. So you'll stay on it until you reach your target.
- It offers a 'sliding-scale' system of diets that you move down through as you lose weight, so there's no plateau.

While you are speed slimming, you will also be achieving the body *shape* you want, with the twelve-minutes-a-day shaping routine, plus optional exercise supplements for your own particular shape problems.

And once that weight is off? There's a good weight-maintenance programme that will help you stay slim for life. Staying Slim, Chapter 10, will show you how to build your own life-long eating plan, based on the good eating habits you will have acquired on the diet. My new and exclusive Food Charts (page 126) will give you the at-a-glance back-up you'll need in order to control your fat and carbohydrate intake. You'll be pleased to hear you need never count calories again; you can slim and *stay* slim on the Complete Speed Slimming System. Start now! You'll be glad you did.

1 Speed Slimming: How It Will Work For You

Nine out of ten people who want to lose weight want to lose it quickly. Yet time and time again we've been told that the only 'sensible' way to lose weight is slowly – at about a pound or so a week. In one, vital way this theory is false, because when we see the weight coming off this slowly we simply give up the fight and choose to stay as we are.

The fact is that *fast, regular* weight loss *right down to our target weight* keeps us motivated. Actually seeing results in the mirror and on the scales is the great driving force that keeps our weight-loss campaign going.

So, the very good news is that you *can* slim quickly – without feeling guilty. It is possible to eat plenty, eat sensibly, feel and look healthy, *and* lose weight fast – all of which can be achieved on the Complete Speed Slimming System.

My Complete Speed Slimming System depends in no way upon very low-calorie, 'crash' or fad diets to work – most of you will be eating *more* than you would on most other weight-loss programmes. There is absolutely no need to exist on a diet of lettuce leaves or meagre portions of food in order to see fast results.

The Complete Speed Slimming System works, not by asking you to eat next to nothing, but in the opposite way, by *increasing* your metabolic rate so that you burn up calories faster – at or near your own potential maximum.

Your metabolic rate is the rate at which your body uses up energy (fuel; in other words calories) in order to function and carry out its work. Your body's source of this energy is the calories in the food and drink that you consume. And, although, for example, the *average* woman is supposed to use up about 1940 calories in energy every day, and the *average* man 2550, some people will need much more than this and some much less. Put simply, you can give one woman an average day's menu and she will use up all the calories in that food in the course of one day, and perhaps she'll still require more. If these additional calories aren't forthcoming by way of more food or drink, she will have to use up the existing fat stores within her body for energy. This woman has a higher-than-average metabolic rate and is likely to be slim.

Give exactly the same day's menu to another woman and she may not use up all the calories in that food. The surplus calories will be converted into body fat. This woman has a lower-than-average metabolic rate and is likely to put on weight unless she eats less, or finds ways to use up more calories – and thus speed up her metabolism.

There are various ways in which you can greatly increase your metabolic rate – the rate at which you burn up calories – and this is where the Complete Speed Slimming System comes in. It offers you a reduced-calorie diet (as opposed to a very low-calorie diet), while incorporating every *single way* I know of, to speed up your metabolic rate – and keep the weight moving off fast. Here are the ways to do it:

Through What and How You Eat

• A high-carbohydrate diet

The food that you eat provides you with calories from three types of food – fat, carbohydrate and protein. We now know that if you eat a diet rich in carbohydrates – particularly the natural complex carbohydrates like potatoes, pasta, bread and cereals, rice, pulses, fruits and vegetables – while at the same time eating a diet low in saturated (animal) fat – your metabolic rate speeds up. This means that you can eat more calories on a high complex-carbohydrate diet and lose weight at the same rate as if you ate a lower-calorie diet higher in fat and low in carbohydrates.

Research indicates that this increased metabolic activity is equivalent to anything up to 300 calories a day. This means that on a high-carbohydrate, low-fat diet of around 1300 calories a day you should lose weight at the same rate as on a low-carbohydrate, higher-fat diet of 1000 calories a day. Those 300 calories are equivalent to one complete average dieter's meal!

Or, rather than allowing yourself more food to make up for that 300-calorie difference, you could, for example, eat 1000 calories a day of high-carbohydrate foods and you would lose weight *more quickly* than someone eating 1000 calories a day of low-carbohydrate foods.

The reason for this metabolism-boosting effect appears to be that carbohydrate calories are less easily converted into fat; your body actually prefers to use them as fuel, rather than store them. Dietary fat, however, is very easily converted to body fat, and if there are any excess calories in your diet, it's the fat that will appear on your body first.

Protein can't be turned into fat by your body – it is used either to build, repair or replace the body tissues such as muscle; or as an energy source; any excess is excreted by the body.

So, the ideal slimming diet – and the one incorporated into the Complete Speed Slimming System – is a very high-carbohydrate diet, with very few calories eaten in the form of fat, and with just enough protein for our needs.

An ideal balance in a slimming diet is:

Fat (no more than half of your fat intake should be in the form of saturated [animal] fats)	20%
Carbohydrates	65 – 70%
Protein	10 – 15%

The seventy per cent carbohydrates should ideally be completely made up of complex carbohydrates, as explained above. There is another type of carbohydrate – 'simple' carbohydrates, which are basically sugar in its various forms, and alcohol. These simple carbohydrates currently form a large part of our diet in the Western world and we should try to eat less of them. While these simple carbohydrates are an easily converted source of energy, they actually have no nutritional value. So the calories they offer are 'empty', so to speak, and your nutritional needs will have to be met by other foods, which will only add to your calorie intake. The World Health Organisation (WHO) suggests the upper limit of simple carbohydrate consumption should be ten per cent – so the Complete Speed Slimming System allows for between five and ten per cent of your total calorie intake in the form of simple carbohydrates. This still allows for up to sixty-five per cent of your total calories to be eaten in the form of complex carbohydrates; together they provide a total carbohydrate level ideal to achieve maximum metabolism increase.

There are, by the way, other advantages to a complex-carbohydrate rich diet: better digestion and elimination; a feeling of fullness so there are no hunger pangs or problems with willpower. These are the benefits people have experienced when following the Complete Speed Slimming principles.

• The snacking system

Frequent eating is another key to raising your metabolism. Again, you could eat 1000 calories a day all in one big meal, and you would lose weight *more slowly* than if you eat your 1000 calories in five small meals. The increased metabolic activity caused by snacking can be up to 100 extra calories a day.

This is because the act of eating takes energy. Think of frequent eating as keeping your metabolic fires 'stoked' and on the go all the time. The other advantage of snack eating when you are slimming is that it helps to keep the hunger pangs at bay, and because it provides your body with manageable quantities, expended as needed, it is an eating pattern that your digestive system prefers.

• Other food factors

Other, more minor, food factors can also affect the rate at which you burn up calories. Research indicates that a diet high in raw foods, in cold foods, in vitamin C and in spices such as ginger and chilli can speed up your metabolism. The total combined effect of these added food factors could mean a speed-up factor equivalent of fifty calories a day, or more in many cases.

THROUGH THE RIGHT EXERCISE PLAN

• Low-intensity aerobic work

You can burn off an extra 400 calories a day just by doing an hour's aerobic activity. This means burning up to 300 calories during the actual process of exercising, and up to 100 calories equivalent increase in metabolic rate during the next twenty-four hours! In other words, if you exercise aerobically every day, your metabolic rate will be permanently increased, even when you are asleep!

Low-intensity aerobic work is a fairly gentle level of exercise that anyone can do, and the system pioneered in this book is a safe one, ensuring that you can work out aerobically even if your current fitness level is poor.

• Strength and tone exercise

The body shaping plans in Chapter 9 help improve your metabolic rate as well as your shape by increasing your body's proportion of lean tissue (muscle) as you lose fat. Lean tissue is more metabolically active than fat; i.e., it is very active tissue that needs to be provided with energy to sustain it; unlike fat, which is fairly inactive.

For more information on the way exercise helps increase your metabolism and encourage your slimming campaign, turn to Chapters 8 and 9.

THROUGH YOUR LIFESTYLE

• Get plenty of fresh air

A speedy metabolism simply means that you are burning off more calories. To burn them off, your body needs oxygen; therefore, to help things along, you should get as much fresh air as you can, and learn how to breathe more deeply throughout your everyday life. Sleep with an open window; if you work in centrally heated offices you must make an effort to get regular fresh air. You should also ensure that you don't live permanently in an overheated atmosphere. Your metabolism will slow down if it doesn't have to work hard to keep you warm. Over-warmth can lead to a sluggish feeling, which means you'll be less likely to take on anything requiring activity.

• Get busy

A couch-potato lifestyle slows down your metabolism. Keep your body active and it will repay you by burning off many extra calories a day. For ideas on how to increase your activity, turn to page 77. You should also consider your sleep pattern; if you regularly get more than eight hours' sleep a night, ask yourself if you *really* need this amount. Half an hour's sleep *less* a night is equivalent to an average of fifty or a hundred extra calories being burned up, depending upon what activity you decide to replace sleep with.

• Stay happy

One final interesting fact is that your body's metabolism slows down when you are depressed, bored or miserable. Laughter, fun and excitement, new challenges and new experiences all speed it up. So don't sit there feeling fed up while you slim – get out and enjoy life!

There is one important factor that sets the Complete Speed Slimming System apart from other diets. This system not only helps you to evaluate your own metabolic rate, and set your calorie level according to the results, but it actually matches your diet to the amount of weight you need to lose.

THE SLIDING-SCALE DIETS

Most diet plans totally ignore the fact that the more weight you have to lose, the more you should be eating on your diet. Simply speaking, this is because the more overweight you are, the more you have been eating to maintain that weight. A woman of, say, fourteen stone (88.9 kg) who should weigh nearer to nine stone (57.2 kg) may have been eating about 3000 calories a day to maintain that weight. If she starts dieting at 1500 calories a day, she will have a daily 'deficit' of 1500 calories. The deficit will be large enough to produce excellent weight loss at the start of her diet. As she slims down, however, she will need to slowly reduce the calories in the diet in order to continue experiencing that swift weight loss.

In the same way, a woman who only needs to lose a stone or so will need to *begin* dieting on slightly fewer calories. And that is what the Complete Speed Slimming System does for everyone – it decides your correct dieting level at any given time and moves you down through a sliding scale of diets so that there is *no plateau*. And, because people who need to eat more *are* eating more, there is never a problem of hunger for long-term dieters. Lastly, because each of the sliding-scale diets is slightly different, with different menus and new recipes, you won't become bored.

THE METABOLISM ASSESSMENT

Because one of the main assets of the Complete Speed Slimming System is that you'll raise your metabolic rate, it is important to assess whether your own existing rate is high, average or low. This is done through a detailed personal assessment in Chapter 3. Depending upon the results, you then follow a diet plan that is slightly amended to fit your individual circumstances.

In all there are *fifteen* different dieting options available to slimmers on the Complete Speed Slimming System. In Chapter 3 you will be guided easily and quickly to the correct diet that will get *you* down to your target weight as quickly as possible!

Fast Weight Loss: All Your Questions Answered

2

Tens of thousands of people have slimmed successfully following the methods outlined in this book. This next section covers all the questions most frequently asked both about the Complete Speed Slimming System and about fast weight loss in general.

What are the benefits of losing weight quickly?

Surveys show that the main reason people give up on diets – or never begin them – is a combination of boredom and lack of visible results. One to two pounds a week hardly shows; three or more *does*. In other words, people need motivation to stay on a weight-loss diet, and motivation is not inspired by slow results.

Secondly, there is more to life than dieting; and people have more important things to do than constantly monitor a semi-permanent and slow weight loss diet. The best way to lose weight is to realise that nothing can be achieved if you do it half-heartedly. You *will* succeed if you apply the same determination and effort to this as you would to any other problem affecting your life.

What puts some people *off* the idea of fast weight loss is that they believe they will only be allowed to eat a little in order to succeed, thus bringing superhuman willpower and awful hunger pangs into the picture. However, with the Complete Speed Slimming System, this does not happen; you need never be hungry.

If fast weight loss is safe, why has crash dieting acquired such a bad name over the years?

Crash dieting is not one and the same as fast weight loss. Crash dieting conjures up images of fad diets that are very low in calories, and, in turn, poor nutrition. Crash dieting – on, say, less than 800 calories a day short-term or 1000 calories a day long term – usually means that your diet will be short of many essential nutrients, vitamins and minerals needed for a healthy body. That is even more likely if the crash diet is a fad diet, relying on only one or two foods; e.g., the egg and grapefruit diet, or the cheese and tomato diet. These are the diets that, quite rightly, have a bad name and I would advise you to steer well clear of them.

Crash dieting is not an advisable way to slim. The Complete Speed Slimming System is *not* a crash or fad diet and does not ask you to eat like a bird. It relies on reducing the calories *a little* and on speeding up your metabolic rate. The diets contain as many calories as you will eat on any other healthy slimming diet – and sometimes more.

If you follow the Complete Speed Slimming System, you will be eating plenty and re-educating your eating habits so that, with the help of the maintenance programme in Chapter 10, you won't ever put the weight back on. So if you have been a 'yo-yo' dieter – or are perhaps worried that you might be one – with the apparent risks to your health that such a regime brings, you need have no fears.

Fast weight loss, carried out correctly, is *safe*.

However few calories I eat, I still find it really hard to lose weight. Will your method work for me?

Assuming you don't have a hormonal problem (i.e., thyroid, and very few people do), then if you follow the instructions and complete all the questionnaires in the Complete Speed Slimming System, you will find it a lot easier to lose weight than on any other diet I can think of. The reasons for this are detailed throughout this chapter.

Failure to lose weight on a diet usually comes down to one of two things: you are either eating more than you think you are – dare I say cheating? – (and the diet plans in this book help you to avoid that by providing you with plenty to eat) or, the diet does not contain a suitable calorie level for your specific needs. The Complete Speed Slimming System, however, ensures that you *do* match your calorie levels to your individual needs and metabolic rate. So be sure to give it your best effort.

Is the Complete Speed Slimming System safe for anyone of any age?

Because the diets in this book are sensible and healthy, and because the exercise plan is carefully graded according to your fitness, this system is safe for any adult in good health who needs to lose weight. However, if you are under eighteen, over sixty-five, pregnant, breastfeeding, or suffering or convalescing from any chronic illness, I would advise you not to start on this or any other diet plan without your doctor's knowledge and full consent, so check with him or her first.

Why do you think that the Complete Speed Slimming System is better than other quick-loss diets; for example, the formula shake mixes?

One objection I have to the low-calorie shake mixes as a form of dieting is that they take no account of the important fact that the more weight you have to lose, the more calories you should eat. An eighteen-stone (114.3 kg) man who wants to lose six stone (38.1 kg) will be eating the same paltry 600 calories or so a day as a ten-stone (63.5 kg) woman who wants to lose a stone (6.4 kg). Also, as explained above, very-low-calorie levels just aren't necessary. There is also the boredom factor of these shake diets as well as the fact that they are *not* high in complex carbohydrates, which are necessary to speed up your metabolism. And, of course, drinking a milkshake (or eating a biscuit bar) three times a day throughout your diet does not help you to understand what a really balanced and healthy diet is; so when the time comes to maintain your weight, you may flounder.

Finally, in 1987 an official government report on very-low-calorie meal-replacement type diets stated quite clearly that they shouldn't be used for people with only a little weight to lose; that they shouldn't be used long-term as a sole source of nutrition (therefore limiting their use for people with a *lot* of weight to lose); and should not be used until 'real food' diets had been tried.

Doesn't fast weight loss mean that you lose muscle tissue rather than fat?

On any slimming diet, a certain amount of the overall weight that you lose will be matter other than fat. This is true whether you lose weight quickly or slowly. The allegation that more lean tissue is lost on a fast weight-loss diet was made in the early 1980s by a Royal College of Physicians' report on obesity. Since then, however, no fewer than five separate independent trials have proved that the percentage of lean tissue lost is more dependent upon a person's own genes and predisposition to lean tissue loss than on any other factor, and that the *speed* of weight loss is *not* a factor.

Even more significant perhaps are the findings of a trial conducted by the well-respected Dunn Nutrition Unit at Cambridge. In this trial, the lean body tissue masses of a group of dieters who had achieved their 'correct' weight were compared to those of a group of people of the same sex and weight who had never dieted. The results were almost identical.

On the Complete Speed Slimming System you will be *building* lean muscle tissue through the fat burning and body shaping routines.

You say that the Complete Speed Slimming System makes you burn up calories faster, but I thought that dieting made you fat by slowing down your metabolic rate.

The idea behind this theory is that when you diet, your body has a reaction mechanism; it thinks you are starving it, and therefore, to conserve energy, it slows down its metabolic rate so that it burns calories more slowly. The more you diet, this idea went, the slower your metabolism would become and the harder it would be to shed pounds.

This 'starvation mode' theory is no longer

regarded as true. In fact, to my knowledge, the only trials that have been carried out on this subject were done by the Dunn Nutrition Centre at Cambridge. They found that women dieters, who had slimmed down to the same weight as women who had not been dieting, had metabolic rates similar to the always-slim, non-dieting women.

What *is* true, however, is that, all other factors being equal, your own personal metabolic rate will be slower at the end of a weight-loss diet than it was at the start. How much slower depends on the amount of weight you have lost, since the heavier you are, the higher your metabolic rate. At, say, twelve stone (76.7 kg), you would burn up more calories in your everyday activities than you would at, say, nine stone (57.2 kg). The reason for this is that the heavier you are, the more work your body has to do in moving itself around. In the same way that you would expend more energy in lifting two bags of shopping up a flight of stairs than in lifting just one bag, so your body would use more calories 'lifting' a twelve-stone (76.7 kg) weight around than a nine-stone (57.2 kg) weight.

That is why, as I keep saying, a heavier person can still lose weight while eating more calories than a slimmer person. This is why on the Complete Speed Slimming System I ask you to re-assess your calorie intake at regular intervals in order to maintain a good rate of weight loss.

The Complete Speed Slimming System goes a long way towards counteracting the effects of the natural metabolism-slowing process because whilst you are dieting, you are at the same time practising ways to *boost* your metabolism. If you follow all the suggestions for lifestyle modifications as well as the diet and exercise programme, you could end up at your target weight with a metabolic rate equivalent to, or in some cases higher than, what it was when you were at your heaviest weight.

Once you have reached your target weight, what you have to remember is that you began putting on weight in the first place because you were probably eating more calories than your body needed for energy each day. If you go back to your old eating habits you will put weight on again. This isn't because 'dieting makes you fat' – it is because eating more than you need for your own requirements makes you fat.

Won't I feel hungry on a fast weight-loss diet?
On some diets you may, but not on this one. The Complete Speed Slimming System contains plenty of high-carbohydrate, high-fibre foods which fill you up and help you to feel full for longer. And you will be eating at least four times a day, so you'll never have to go for long periods without food. The calorie content of the diets is not too low, and it is matched to how much weight *you* need to lose and to *your own* metabolism – so you won't ever have to diet on a level that's not right for your own needs. If you have a lot of weight to lose, you will be surprised at just how much you *can* eat when you begin the diet.

What will happen if I follow the diet without doing the exercise plans?
You will still lose weight, but you will not lose it as quickly. The calorie and fat burning effects of the routines outlined in Chapter 8, and the lean-tissue-building effects of the routines in Chapter 9, have a great influence on your metabolism and the speed at which you lose those unwanted pounds. Also, as your body's metabolism naturally slows down, as you eat less and less, it is important to boost it as much as you can.

Unless you have a medical reason, I would not advise you to diet without exercising, because of all the additional benefits that exercise brings – tone and shape, fitness and well-being, to name just a few. If your reason for not exercising is anything other than medical, you must ask yourself why you don't want to exercise. Many people cite lack of time; if this is your problem, sit down with pen and paper and write out everything you do during your waking hours over, say, a week. Frankly assess whether or not any specific activity is more important than keeping (or getting) your body fit and slim?

Remember, unlike more dispensable items like your car, your body cannot be changed for a newer model when it gets rusty or gives trouble. It deserves your time and attention. It is sometimes difficult to accept that it is not selfish for you to make time for yourself and your body. So even if your schedule is busy because you are always working or caring for others, try to make time for yourself.

One other reason people often don't want to embark upon an exercise programme is that they think it will be painful, or too difficult. This programme takes care of those problems by giving you an individual fitness assessment, and by making sure that you start on a level that is suitable for you. It also requires you to exercise within sensible limits and it never asks you to compare your progress with another person's. Maybe you won't, for instance, be able to perform some of the body shaping exercises fully to start with, but after a few weeks – in some cases even a few days – of limbering up, and trying your best (without hurting yourself), you really will be surprised at what you can do.

Why do so many experts tell us to lose weight very slowly and gradually?

The main theory behind this is that while losing weight slowly you are re-educating your eating patterns and your appetite. Also, many so-called experts still believe that fast weight loss is unsafe – confusing safe forms of losing weight quickly with bad, mad, crash, very-low-calorie diets.

The Complete Speed Slimming System takes great care to provide all slimmers with a healthy, balanced, sensible diet of varied foods – the same foods that will form your maintenance diet once you've lost weight.

What you must remember is that many nutritionists, doctors and dietitians obtained their qualifications a long time ago, and perhaps haven't kept up to date with the latest research. Many experts I meet in the course of my work still quote the 'dieting makes you fat' and 'dieting loses lean tissue' theories popular ten years ago; even though the weight of evidence today now shows they are false and should be disregarded.

Isn't it true that weight lost quickly comes back even more quickly?

I do believe that if you lose weight – quickly or slowly – on a fad diet relying on only a few types of food or on meal replacements, then you will have no idea how to eat to maintain your new weight when you end the diet. You will probably go back to your old eating habits, and the weight will come back on.

A good diet will teach you how you should be eating and will also offer long-term advice on controlling eating problems – binges, comfort eating, coping with your social life, and so on. No scientific evidence or trials conducted in the past show that weight lost quickly comes back just as quickly. Nor is there any truth in the idea that after a weight-reducing diet you have to exist on a 'dieting' level of calories for the rest of your life.

One very important reason that many people do put weight back on is that they lose their motivation to stay slim. Once you have achieved something, motivation can often disappear.

So how will the Complete Speed Slimming System help me to stay slim afterwards?

This system will gradually build up your calorie intake after you have reached target so that your dieting period doesn't just suddenly stop – it 'evolves' into the maintenance period. It is a continuing diet, comprised of the kinds of food you have been eating while you have been losing weight – so there is no sudden change in that direction, either. You simply eat *more* of the things you've been eating on your diet, plus some additional extras. It offers simple solutions to ongoing eating problems, and advice to help you maintain your higher metabolic rate so that you can eat plenty on your maintenance diet without putting on an ounce.

If you lose weight and then put it all back on, isn't it even harder to lose weight the next time you try?

This relates to the 'dieting makes you fat' theory, popular in some quarters, that every time you diet, you lose more and more 'lean tissue', which is replaced by fat tissue. In fact, this doesn't happen. Probably the only reason that people who have lost and then regained weight find it harder to diet the second time is psychological. However, if you follow the Complete Speed Slimming System, weight gain is unlikely and so the question won't arise.

How fast will I lose weight on the Complete Speed Slimming System?

If you follow all the instructions and metabolism-boosting methods in the book, I can assure you that you will lose weight more quickly on this system than on any other diet with a similar calorie content. It isn't possible to predict exactly how many pounds you will lose in a week. What I can tell you is that you will lose approximately five to seven pounds (2.3 – 3.2 kg) the first week of dieting, and after that approximately three to four pounds (1.4 – 1.8 kg) a week throughout most of your diet.

The reason you lose more weight in the first week is that you are losing glycogen, a mixture of glucose and water that is stored in the liver as instant energy. It is depleted when you reduce your food intake, before you begin to burn off fat tissue.

3 How Much Weight Do You Need To Lose?

The diets in Chapter 5 will form the core of your weight-loss programme. This programme has been specially designed to fit *your* particular needs, and that's why it works. Whoever you are, and however much or little you need to lose; however hard you've found it to stick to slimming plans before; however slowly you've seen the weight come off before ... *this* one *will* work for *you*.

Everything you need for your own personal diet campaign is here, so you'll slim quickly, easily and without pain!

There are five interlinking diet plans (and a *speed plus* short-term diet for special use; that is explained fully on page 55). The more weight you have to lose, the greater the number of these plans you will follow. The more you have to lose, the more you can eat – and still lose weight quickly. As you get nearer your target weight you'll reduce the amount you eat in order to keep up the weight loss at a steady rate.

The five diet plans start off with *Diet 1*, with a calorie intake 'high' of up to 1500 calories a day, going down gradually to *Diet 5*, which helps you to lose those last few pounds on between 900 and 1000 calories a day. Moving from diet to diet also helps prevent boredom setting in – and that's death to even the best dieting intentions!

The Complete Speed Slimming Diet Programme incorporates not only this sliding-scale format to help speed up and maintain your weight loss, but it also incorporates *all* the tried and tested ways to speed up your own personal metabolic rate (the rate at which your body uses energy [the calories in your food]). Through this you can increase your rate of weight loss *without* the need to crash diet.

Here are the keys to weight loss the Complete Speed Slimming System way.

- You will be eating a diet high in complex carbohydrates – bread, potatoes, rice, pasta, pulses, fruit and vegetables – and low in fat. Remember, it's not just how much you eat that is vital to weight loss and good health, but what you eat.
- You spread your calorie intake fairly evenly throughout the day, eating an average of four or five times a day. The snacking principle burns off extra calories!
- The diet is rich in Vitamin C, and raw and spicy foods, all of which help to keep your metabolism ticking over well.
- The diet helps stave off the 'slimming blues' – the hunger pangs, headaches, lethargy and general misery that other boring, tasteless, low-calorie dieting regimes can bring.

All these methods, combined with the wonderful metabolism-boosting effects you will be getting by following the Complete Speed Slimming exercise routines, will help you to achieve the fast and easy weight loss you've always wanted.

YOUR WEIGHT-LOSS TARGET

Before you begin the programme, you must complete the following weight loss analysis to discover which of the five diet plans you should start on. Do this even if you *think* you already know how much weight you need to lose.

There are various ways to ascertain how much weight you need to lose: height/weight charts, the Body Mass Index (BMI), and your previous 'normal' weight (if you have ever been there) will all help to guide you.

The best system for working out your correct target weight is a combination of several ways. So follow this step-by-step guide, and at the end you should have a virtually fool-proof correct target and expected weight loss.

Test 1. Apply Some Common Sense

If you have gained most of your excess weight in your adult years, can you remember the last weight at which you felt 'good', as an adult?

If so, write it here:

.... st .... lbs (......... kg)

If you were at this weight a very long time ago (i.e., you were in your twenties and you're now in your fifties), it is probably more sensible to aim for a weight about seven pounds (3.2 kg) higher, at least to start with. You can always re-assess. If you want to adjust your normal target, do so here:

.... st .... lbs (......... kg)

If you have never been slim as an adult, but have an idea of what you would *like* to weigh, write it here:

.... st .... lbs (......... kg)

If you have *never* been slim as an adult and have no idea at all of what you should weigh, leave the above spaces blank and move on.

Test 2. Use the Height/Weight Chart

Most of you will have filled in some kind of target weight above. Now we have to apply some science to see if, indeed, this is a suitable target weight for you. For this you must use the height/weight charts overleaf.

It is sensible to be wary of height/weight charts in general, because they can vary enormously. Some give just one specific target to aim for, while other charts have widely differing views about what is a sensible lower and upper weight range.

The chart I have devised is, I think, an excellent compromise between the various figures floating around. It is in part based on the Royal College of Physicians' chart, but I have raised their lower limits slightly in accordance with more recent advice.

Look at the chart and find your height. Does the final weight you wrote in at the end of Test 1 fall within the upper and lower limits given?

YES ☐ NO ☐ DON'T KNOW ☐

If you answered yes, and your target weight is neither right on the lower or upper limit, you can safely assume that it is a good weight for you. You can, however, try Test 3 if you wish to double-check. If you have seven pounds (3.2 kg) or less to lose, you should also carry out Tests 4, 5 and 6 just to be sure.

If you answered yes, but your target weight is at or very near the *maximum* given for your height, that's probably fine, but you should continue to Test 3 as a further check. Once you have reached your target you should do a re-assessment by answering Tests 4, 5 and 6 to see if you need to lose any more weight.

If you answered yes, but your target weight is at or very near the *minimum* given for your height, that's also probably all right. But you should undertake Test 3 as a further check, and once you have slimmed down to within seven pounds (3.2 kg) of your target weight, you should come back to this section and complete Tests 4, 5 and 6 before deciding whether you really do need to lose any more weight.

If, however, you target weight is at or very near the *minimum* given, and you only need to lose seven pounds (3.2 kg) or less now, then you should answer Tests 3, 4, 5 and 6 *before* you begin to diet.

If you answered no, and your target weight at the end of Test 1 is outside the upper or lower limits given in the height/weight charts, then proceed as follows: If your target was *lower*, adjust your target weight to the *minimum* figure given and proceed as above. If your target weight was *higher*, it may be OK, but you should proceed to Test 3 and do the Body Mass Index (BMI) check.

If you didn't know the answer to Test 1 (i.e., you couldn't manage to find a target weight for you) you can proceed as follows: If you have more than two stone (12.7 kg) to lose, choose a target weight at or near the *maximum* ideal weight given for your height. For example, if you are five feet five inches (1.60 m) tall and currently weight twelve

HEIGHT/WEIGHT CHART FOR WOMEN

(Height without shoes; weight without clothes)

HEIGHT	MINIMUM ACCEPTABLE WEIGHT	MAXIMUM ACCEPTABLE WEIGHT
4 ft 10 ins (1.45 m)	7 st 1 lb (45 kg)	8 st 10 lbs (55 kg)
4 ft 11 ins (1.48 m)	7 st 3 lbs (46 kg)	8 st 12 lbs (56 kg)
5 ft 0 ins (1.50 m)	7 st 5 lbs (47 kg)	9 st 0 lbs (57 kg)
5 ft 1 in (1.52 m)	7 st 7 lbs (48 kg)	9 st 3 lbs (59 kg)
5 ft 2 ins (1.54 m)	7 st 10 lbs (49 kg)	9 st 6 lbs (60 kg
5 ft 3 ins (1.56 m)	7 st 13 lbs (50 kg)	9 st 9 lbs (61 kg)
5 ft 4 ins (1.58 m)	8 st 2 lbs (52 kg)	9 st 12 lbs (63 kg)
5 ft 5 ins (1.60 m)	8 st 6 lbs (54 kg)	10 st 2 lbs (65 kg)
5 ft 6 ins (1.62 m)	8 st 10 lbs (55 kg)	10 st 6 lbs (66 kg)
5 ft 7 ins (1.64 m)	9 st 0 lbs (57 kg)	10 st 10 lbs (68 kg)
5 ft 8 ins (1.66 m)	9 st 4 lbs (59 kg)	11 st 2 lbs (71 kg)
5 ft 9 ins (1.68 m)	9 st 8 lbs (61 kg)	11st 6 lbs (73 kg)
5 ft 10 ins (1.70 m)	9 st 12 lbs (63 kg)	11st 10 lbs (75 kg)
5 ft 11 ins (1.72 m)	10 st 2 lbs (65 kg)	12 st 0 lbs (76 kg)
6 ft 0 ins (1.74 m)	10 st 6 lbs (66 kg)	12 st 4 lbs (78 kg)

HEIGHT/WEIGHT CHART FOR MEN

(Height without shoes; weight without clothes)

HEIGHT	MINIMUM ACCEPTABLE WEIGHT	MAXIMUM ACCEPTABLE WEIGHT
5 ft 2 ins (1.54 m)	8 st 9 lbs (55 kg)	10 st 6 lbs (66 kg)
5 ft 3 ins (1.56 m)	8 st 12 lbs (56 kg)	10 st 9 lbs (68 kg)
5 ft 4 ins (1.58 m)	9 st 1 lb (58 kg)	10 st 12 lbs (68 kg)
5 ft 5 ins (1.60 m)	9 st 4 lbs (59 kg)	11 st 2 lbs (71 kg)
5 ft 6 ins (1.62 m)	9 st 8 lbs (61 kg)	11 st 5 lbs (72 kg)
5 ft 7 ins (1.64 m)	9 st 12 lbs (63 kg)	11 st 8 lbs (74 kg)
5 ft 8 ins (1.66 m)	10 st 2 lbs (65 kg)	12 st 0 lbs (76 kg)
5 ft 9 ins (1.68 m)	10 st 6 lbs (66 kg)	12 st 6 lbs (79 kg)
5 ft 10 ins (1.70 m)	10 st 10 lbs (68 kg)	12 st 10 lbs (81 kg)
5 ft 11 ins (1.72 m)	11 st 0 lbs (70 kg)	13 st 0 lbs (83 kg)
6 ft 0 ins (1.74 m)	11 st 4 lbs (72 kg)	13 st 6 lbs (85 kg)
6 ft 1 in (1.76 m)	11 st 8 lbs (74 kg)	13 st 11 lbs (88 kg)
6 ft 2 ins (1.78 m)	11 st 13 lbs (76 kg)	14 st 2 lbs (90 kg)
6 ft 3 ins (1.80 m)	12 st 4 lbs (78 kg)	14 st 7 lbs (92 kg)
6 ft 4 ins (1.82 m)	12 st 9 lbs (80 kg)	14 st 12 lbs (95 kg)

stone seven pounds (79.4 kg), then you should aim initially for ten stone two pounds (64.4 kg). When you reach that target, you can re-assess yourself by returning and answering Tests 4, 5 and 6.

If you have less than two stone (12.7 kg) to lose, but your current weight is still higher than the *maximum* ideal weight given for your height, then aim for a target weight somewhere between the minimum and the maximum. For example, if you are five feet five inches (1.60m) tall and you currently weigh eleven stone (69.9 kg), aim for a target weight of around nine stone two or three pounds (58.1 – 58.5kg). As you get near your target, re-assess by answering Tests 4, 5 and 6.

If your current weight is *lower* than the *maximum* ideal weight given – for example, you weigh nine stone eight pounds (60.8 kg) at five feet five inches (1.60 m) – you should answer Tests 3, 4, 5 and 6 before beginning a diet. You may not need to lose any weight at all.

After consulting the height/weight charts and following the instructions in Test 2, my target weight is:

.... st .... lbs (......... kg)

This weight may be the same as your target weight at the end of the first section.

Test 3. Your Body Mass Index (BMI)

The Body Mass Index (BMI) is a different way of assessing your correct target weight without using height/weight charts. Work out the BMI for your target weight as follows:

- Convert your target weight into kilos (divide the number of pounds by 2.2).
- Convert your height into metres (multiply the number of inches by 0.025).

  Alternatively, look at the height weight charts (opposite) where approximate metric equivalents are given.
- Now, using a calculator, square your height (e.g., 1.8 m × 1.8 m).
- Now divide your target weight by your squared height. The resulting figure is what your BMI will be if you reach your chosen target weight.

If your answer falls anywhere between 20 and 25, you have chosen a weight that is considered to be suitable for you. Under 20 and you're aiming too low, over 25 and your target weight may be too high. If your BMI is between 26 and 29 you are considered clinically overweight.

Example

Your target weight is 9 stone, which is 126 lbs.

$\frac{126}{2.2}$ = 57.3 kg (57 kg to round it off).

Your height is 5 ft 5 ins, which is 65ins.

$65 \times 0.025 = 1.63$ m.

$1.63 \times 1.63 = 2.65$

$\frac{57}{2.65}$ = 21.5. Rounded off, this is 21.

Your answer, then is 21.

For interest's sake, work out your current BMI (at the weight you are now). If it is between 30 and 40, you are clinically obese. If it is over 40, you are severely obese.

Obviously, if you have a severe weight problem it is better to aim for a BMI of about 26 or 27, than to remain at 35. If your target BMI works out at 26, don't aim lower for now. The best thing is to get to 26 and then re-asses yourself. If your target BMI is lower than 20, however, adapt it to fall within the range. There is absolutely no point in becoming too slim. Fill in the following:

My target BMI is ....

My current BMI is ....

My target weight is .... st .... lbs (......... kg)

(For many people this will still be the same as at the end of Tests 1 and 2.)

If the results of Tests 1, 2 and 3 indicate that you have a lot of weight to lose, it is probably not worth completing Tests 4, 5 and 6 until you are nearer your target weight. But if you have seven pounds or less to lose, or your target weight or BMI is at or near the *minimum* acceptable, then proceed with Tests 4, 5 and 6. You should also come back and use them to re-assess your target weight when you are within seven pounds of reaching it.

Test 4. Take Your Measurements

Woman readers, measure your hips around their widest part. Check this measurement against the height/hip chart that follows. If your hips are the same or smaller than the measurement given, you probably don't need to lose any (or more) weight. If they are larger, then you probably do.

Male readers, measure your waist, and check with the height/waist chart below.

Test 5. Look in a Mirror

Wearing just a pair of briefs, stand in front of a full-length mirror and look at yourself from the side and from the front. Ask yourself honestly if you *really* look overweight? Can you pinch extra flesh on your waist, thighs and upper arms? Wiggle around a bit; shake out your legs and arms. Do you still want to lose weight? Don't forget that when you lose weight, you tend to lose it from all over your body; you can't really choose which places to lose it from. So, if you're happy with most of your body, but certain parts of it are worrying you, perhaps your answer is toning and aerobic exercise, like the plans in Chapters 4 and 5. Rolls of fat are one thing, but a flabby, 'loose' feeling to your body may just mean that you're lacking muscle tone. A *shape* that disappoints you rather than a *weight* that disappoints you should always be worked on through exercise.

Text 6. Get Second Opinions

Who can you trust to give you an honest opinion of your size? Your best friend? Your mother? Your

HEIGHT/HIPS RATIO FOR WOMEN

(Measure hips around widest point)

HEIGHT		HIPS SHOULD MEASURE NO MORE THAN	
4 ft 10 ins – 5 ft 0 ins	(1.45 m – 1.50 m)	34 ins	(85 cm)
5 ft 1 in – 5 ft 2 ins	(1.52 m – 1.54 m)	35 ins	(87.5 cm)
5 ft 3 ins – 5 ft 4 ins	(1.56 m – 1.58 m)	36 ins	(90 cm)
5 ft 5 ins – 5 ft 6 ins	(1.60 m – 1.62 m)	37 ins	(92.5 cm)
5 ft 7 ins – 5 ft 8 ins	(1.64 m – 1.66 m)	38 ins	(95 cm)
5 ft 9 ins – 5 ft 10 ins	(1.68 m – 1.70 m)	39 ins	(97.5 cm)
5 ft 11 ins – 6 ft 0 ins	(1.72 m – 1.74 m)	40 ins	(100 cm)

HEIGHT/WAIST RATIO FOR MEN

HEIGHT		WAIST SHOULD MEASURE NO MORE THAN	
5 ft 2 ins – 5 ft 4 ins	(1.54 m – 1.58 m)	30 ins	(75 cm)
5 ft 5 ins – 5 ft 7 ins	(1.60 m – 1.64 m)	31 ins – 32 ins	(77.5 cm – 80 cm)
5 ft 8 ins – 5 ft 10 ins	(1.66 m – 1.70 m)	32 ins – 33 ins	(80 cm – 82.5 cm)
5 ft 11 ins – 6 ft 0 ins	(1.72 m – 1.74 m)	33 ins – 34 ins	(82.5 cm – 85 cm)
6 ft 1 in – 6 ft 2 ins	(1.76 m – 1.78 m)	34 ins – 35 ins	(85 cm – 87.5 cm)
6 ft 3 ins – 6 ft 4 ins	(1.80 m – 1.82 m)	35 ins – 36 ins	(87.5 cm – 90 cm)

husband or daughter? Your colleague? Ask a couple of the people you most trust for their opinion. Consider their answers.

If there is no one you can talk to about this, or if you want yet another opinion, go to your doctor or community dietitian for advice.

If the tests all concur that you don't need to lose any weight and your trusted friend or family member says you don't, you are probably at a weight that is right for you. Eat healthily, go onto the maintenance programme and continue (or start) your exercise programme to achieve the shape you want.

It's important to remember that even if the scales don't register the target weight you had in mind, but you feel and look fine, that is all that matters.

Your Weight Loss Profile

My current weight is:

...12... st ...0... lbs (......... kg)

My target weight is:

...10... st ...13... lbs (......... kg)

The amount of weight I need to lose is:

...1... st ...1... lbs (......... kg)

Check down the following list to find the diet on which you should start.

- *I need to lose more than three stone (19 kg).*
  My starting diet is Diet 1 on page 30.
- *I need to lose between two to three stone (12.7 kg – 19 kg).*
  My starting diet is Diet 2 on page 35.
- *I need to lose between one to two stone (6.4 kg – 12.7 kg).*
  My starting diet is Diet 3 on page 40.
- *I need to lose between eight pounds and one stone (3.6 kg – 6.35 kg).*
  My starting diet is Diet 4 on page 45.
- *I need to lose seven pounds (3.2 kg) or less.*
  My starting diet is Diet 5 on page 49.

So now you know which diet to begin with. But wait, to use this diet to maximum effect, you also need to know your *metabolism profile*. Do you have a high metabolic rate, or is it average or low? We'll discover this through the following six simple questions listed below.

YOUR METABOLISM PROFILE

As I explained in Chapter 1, people with a great deal of weight to lose always have a faster metabolic rate than people with not as much to lose. The sliding-scale diets take that major factor into account. This metabolism profile will assess the factors *other* than your weight which affect your own personal metabolism.

Tick one answer to each question in the boxes provided.

1 Are you:

- Taller than average? ❑ 2
- Of average height? ❑ 1
- Shorter than average? ❑ 0

2 Are you:

- 25 or under? ❑ 2
- 26 – 45? ❑ 1
- Over 45? ❑ 0

3 Are you:

- Naturally slim – never had to diet before? ❑ 2
- Of average build, and muscular? ❑ 1
- Plump, and have been from early childhood? ❑ 0

4 During your average day are you:

- Very active, never sitting still for long? ❑ 2
- Moderately active? ❑ 1
- Sedentary? ❑ 0

5 In your spare time, do you carry out active pursuits (e.g., dancing, walking, cycling, football):

Several times a week or more? ❑ 2

Once or twice a week? ❑ 1

Rarely or never? ❑ 0

6 In terms of your personality, are you:

Excitable, bubbly and happy, getting by on little sleep? ❑ 2

Of average temperament, not too excitable or relaxed? ❑ 1

Calm, quiet, relaxed, never standing when you can sit, and enjoying lots of sleep? ❑ 0

Your Profile

Check through the scores from the boxes you have ticked for each question, and note them here:

1 ......

2 ......

3 ......

4 ......

5 ......

6 ......

The total score is ......

This is your metabolism profile score .

Now select your profile, according to your score.

• If you scored 9 or over

Your metabolic rate is probably higher than for most people of your current weight. Throughout your weight-loss campaign, you will be eating the basic menu *plus* three additional snacks from the choice on page 28. At least two of these snacks should be eaten between breakfast and lunch, or between lunch and your evening meal. The other snack can be eaten *with* a meal. At least one of your snacks should include a fruit.

• If you scored between 4 and 8

Your metabolic rate is probably about average in relation to most people of your current weight. Throughout your weight-loss campaign, you will be eating the basic menus *plus* two additional snacks from the selection on page 28. These snacks should be eaten between breakfast and lunch, and between lunch and your evening meal, and at least one of the snacks should include a fruit.

• If you scored 3 or under

Your metabolic rate is probably low compared to most people of your current weight. Throughout your weight-loss campaign, you will be eating the basic menu *plus* one additional snack from the list on page 28. This snack should be a fruit and it should be eaten mid-afternoon (or mid-morning if you have breakfast very early).

If you are hungry at other times of day, make full use of the *unlimited* list of vegetables on page 29. Nibble on them if you've gone more than about three hours without eating, or if you're feeling too hungry to wait for your next meal. If a meal specifies a dessert, you may also eat this item apart from the meal.

Now you're armed with your weight-loss target, your starting diet and your metabolic profile. All you need to do is read through the following chapter, which includes the general diet instructions and the diets themselves, and you can start to lose that weight.

THE SPEED SLIMMING DIET PROGRAMME

4

The following instructions are extremely important to the Speed Slimming System. Don't skip them! Following these guidelines will ensure you achieve optimum results.

INSTRUCTIONS APPLICABLE TO ALL DIETS

• Now that you know the diet on which you'll begin, all you have to do is stay on it until you reach the lower weight threshold. For example, if you're on Diet 2, with between two and three stone (12.7 kg – 19 kg) to lose, stay on it until you have only two stone (12.7 kg) left to lose. Then move along to the next diet in the book. You then stay on that diet until you reach its lower threshold, and move along the diets until you reach your target weight.

It is vital that once you have reached the lower weight threshold of your current diet, you move along to the next diet. The food intake levels on each diet are appropriate only for that weight-loss target. If you stay on that diet any longer, your weight-loss will inevitably slow down. The next diet will have different meals to choose from, too, so you won't become bored.

• Within Diets 1 to 5 you will find two options: set diets and flexi diets.

The Set Diets

You can choose to follow the set diets where each day's menu is worked out for you in detail so that there are only minimal choices and decisions to make. This is probably a good option for dieters who prefer to be told what to do and who find it difficult to stick to a diet that offers too much choice. If you decide to choose the set diets, simply follow the daily menus (including your snacks, unlimiteds, etc., see pages 28–29). Diets 1 to 4 set out seven daily menus. After seven days simply return to Day 1 again, and repeat the diet as long as is necessary to reach your target weight for that particular diet. Then move on to the next diet on the sliding scale.

The Flexi Diets

The flexi diets are simply a multi-choice option for each diet on the sliding scale. It is up to you to select from the many choices given which breakfast, lunch and evening meal you'll eat. The flexi diet lists appear after the end of the set diets. The flexi diets are probably more suitable if you have particular food needs (i.e., you're a vegetarian), or if there are more than a few foods on the set diets that you don't like.

When following the flexi diets, do make sure to vary your choices as much as possible for maximum nutritional benefit. And don't forget your snacks and unlimiteds (see pages 28–29).

Mix and Match

There is nothing to stop you from using both the set diets and the flexi diets while you slim. Here are some possible combinations:

1 If you have a lot of weight to lose, use the set diet on Diet 1, the flexi diet on Diet 2, the set diet on Diet 3, and so on.

2 Within each diet, you could do the first seven days on the set diet, and then switch to the flexi diet until you have reached the lower weight threshold of that diet.

3 You could even follow the set diet on Day 1, the flexi diet on Day 2, and so on.

There is one thing you *should never do*, and that is to swap from the set diet to the flexi diet *within the same day*.

Check through each day's set diet to make sure all the foods it contains are ones that you enjoy; if they aren't, then follow the flexi diet for the whole of that day.

• **Unlimiteds**. You can freely eat all or any of the items in the lists on page 29 while you diet. It is particularly important to eat plenty from the 'salads' list, so every time 'unlimited salad' is mentioned within your diet, make sure you eat it. It will help fill both you and your plate up, help your meal look more appetising and it will give you vital fibre, vitamins and minerals.

• **Daily allowances**. There is a skimmed milk allowance given for each diet. This is for use in tea or coffee, on cereals where stated, or as a drink on its own.

You need this milk allowance both for the calcium it contains and for the calories. So if you don't drink milk, then you should replace this allowance with either 110 g (4 oz) low-fat natural yoghurt *or* 1 diet fruit yoghurt.

• **Bread**. 'One slice bread' is mentioned frequently within the diets. Unless otherwise stated, this refers to one slice wholemeal bread from a large, medium-cut loaf. If you occasionally choose white bread, granary bread or any other kind of plain bread, your diet won't suffer greatly, but ideally, choose wholemeal. Wholemeal bread contains more fibre, and it will help you to feel full for longer. When French bread is mentioned, that, ideally, should be wholemeal, too.

• **Low-fat spread**. Do not mistake margarines, dairy spreads, sunflower margarines or anything else for low-fat spreads. Any margarine, butter or butter-type spread that doesn't specifically state on its label that it is low- or half-fat is *not* a low-fat spread. Low-fat spreads have half or less than half the calories of other types of fats, so make sure you use them. Hundreds of unwanted calories and fat will be added to your diet if you aren't careful to choose a real low-fat spread.

• **Yoghurts and fromage frais**. Whenever diet yoghurt is listed as an option, you may choose any 125 g (5 oz) pot of fruit yoghurt that contains less than 60 calories a pot (all will be labelled with their calorie content). These 'diet' yoghurts are not the same as ordinary fruit yoghurts labelled 'low-fat'; which may contain up to 135 calories a pot, through their high sugar content.

When the diets offer 'diet' fromage frais, you should be sure to choose one that is specifically a reduced-calorie diet product.

• **Salad dressings**. All dressings should be oil- and fat-free. You can purchase ready-made dressings that fit these requirements (there are lots on offer at the supermarket). Alternatively, you can eat your salads 'undressed', or use lemon juice or plain vinegar (Balsamic vinegar is an excellent choice). When reduced-calorie mayonnaise is mentioned, you can use reduced-calorie salad cream, if you prefer.

• **Planning ahead**. It always helps you to stick to a diet if you plan ahead. Decide what you're going to eat in advance, shop for it, and make sure you have time to prepare it. You'll minimise the chances of cheating. Also, be aware of your own pitfalls. If you don't normally have much time to cook recipe dishes, don't kid yourself that it will all change while you diet. Choose the simpler meal options instead. Select foods that you really enjoy; eat your meals slowly and savour them.

• **Weighing and measuring**. Weighing and measuring has been kept to a minimum wherever possible, but sometimes – especially at the start of your diet – it will be necessary. If you over-estimate quantities of vegetables and fruit, it won't matter as much. But, if you over-estimate your portions of meat, fat, cheese, etc., you could be unwittingly adding hundreds of extra calories to your diet.

After you have been dieting for a while, you will get used to gauging the weights of certain foods by sight. But don't get too complacent about guessing; have a check now and then to make sure you are still accurate.

• **Vegetarians**. If you are vegetarian you may prefer to choose your meals from the flexi diets, where there is a special vegetarian main meal section. But most of the meals on the set diets have a vegetarian option; in fact, the diets are biased towards non-meat meals. When meat is included in a meal, there is usually a vegetarian alternative, and many of the recipe dishes have a meat-free alternative in the footnotes at the end of the recipes.

• **Men**. The Complete Speed Slimming System is just as suitable for men as it is for women. Likewise, male readers should carry out the Weight and Metabolism profiles in Chapter 3 before starting the programme. However, some men, particularly those who are tall or very active, and those with a great deal of weight to lose, may find that they are losing weight so easily that they can add extra foods to their diets.

This can be done in two ways. If you have a low or an average metabolism profile (see pages 23–24), you can simply add one or two extra snacks from the selection offered every day.

If you are already following the high metabolism profile diet, with three extra snacks a day, simply increase portions of these foods by the following amounts, whenever they are mentioned in the diet:

Bread. An extra half slice.
Potatoes. An extra 50 g (2 oz).
Pasta. An extra 15 g (1/2 oz) [dry weight].
Rice. An extra 15 g (1/2 oz) [dry weight].
Meat, poultry or fish. An extra 25 g (1 oz).

If you take either of these options, you may find that as you near target weight, your weight loss slows down, and then you can revert to your original profile.

• **Special cases**. If you are under eighteen, pregnant, breastfeeding, suffering or convalescing from an illness, or elderly, you should obtain your doctor's permission before beginning this or any other reduced-calorie diet.

• **Difficult days**. Every dieter has these, when it seems almost impossible to stick to a diet. Either you have a busy social day, or a work schedule that involves a lot of meetings over meals; or, perhaps you just have an inexplicable urge to eat something that isn't part of the diet.

If this happens to you – and if you're dieting for more than a couple of weeks, you'll have to be a virtual saint and a recluse for it *not* to happen – don't panic. Read Chapter 10 for plenty of advice on how to deal with business and social eating, and apply the same philosophies to your dieting days. To end the day having eaten a *little* more than you should have is much, much better than ending the day having eaten *twice* as much. So if things seem tough, don't use it as an excuse to give up; get straight back on the diet the next day. Or if you know you've eaten a lot more than you should have, turn to page 55 and try the Speed Plus diet for a day or two.

I would also apply the same advice to a sudden urge for a chocolate bar or a slice of cake. If this is a very occasional urge that you don't manage to resist, simply get on with the diet and forget it. The Complete Speed Slimming System is a healthy and filling diet, and most people find that after following it for a few days the urge to binge on sugary, fatty foods will disappear.

If it doesn't, and you do feel the urge to binge, *first* try eating one of the snacks from the list on page 28 (even if it is an extra snack to which you're not normally entitled). There are only around 100 calories in each snack, so they will certainly limit the potential damage. Often the urge to eat something sweet is caused by low blood sugar, and a snack (especially one with fruit) from the lists will quickly ease that.

Once a week you may decide that you wish to indulge in something not on the diet, for example, a chocolate bar, and suffer the slightly lowering rate of weight-loss. In that case, eat it and enjoy it. But if you are the kind of person who doesn't do things by halves, and for whom one chocolate bar at a time is never going to be enough, then I suggest you leave chocolate, or whatever your own particular weakness is, until after you have reached your target weight.

SNACKS

All snacks are approximately 100 calories each. High Mets (those with a high metabolic rate) can choose *three* of these snacks a day, extra to all the meals listed within the diets; Average Mets can choose *two* a day; Low Mets can choose *one* a day.

Choose a snack with fruit for at least one of your daily snacks.

Snacks with Fruit

- Small banana, plus 1 diet fruit yoghurt
- Large banana
- Small fruit (see below for explanations of small and large fruits) plus 2 rye crispbreads with low-fat spread and yeast extract spread (e.g., Marmite)
- Small fruit plus 25g (1 oz) slice malt bread
- Small fruit plus 1 large, plain digestive biscuit
- Small fruit plus can of Weight Watchers low-calorie soup
- Large fruit plus 1 diet fruit yoghurt
- Large fruit plus 1 diet fruit fromage frais
- Large fruit plus 1 rye crispbread spread with 10 g (1/3 oz) vegetable pâté.
- Large fruit plus 1 low-calorie crispbread (e.g., Slymbred) plus 25 g (1 oz) low-fat cottage or soft cheese
- Large fruit plus 1 sachet low-calorie, instant soup
- Large fruit plus 1 sachet low-calorie, instant hot chocolate

Other Snacks

- 1 muesli bar
- 1 Shepherdboy Multi Fruit Bar
- 1 crumpet with a little low-fat spread and 1 tsp pure fruit spread
- 25g (1 oz) salted (or unsalted) unbuttered popcorn
- 25g (1 oz) unsweetened breakfast cereal, with milk from allowance
- 1 slice bread with a little low-fat spread, plain or with a yeast extract spread (e.g., Marmite)
- 25 g (1 oz) dried apricots or peaches plus 1 diet fromage frais or diet yoghurt
- 1 25g (1 oz) bag lower fat crisps

FRUIT

Large Fruit

Choose one item from this list whenever 'large fruit' is mentioned within your diet:

- Apple, 1 medium
- Apple, stewed (using artificial sweetener), 140 g (5 oz)
- Blackberries, stewed (using artificial sweetener), 140 g (5 oz)
- Blackcurrants, stewed (using artificial sweetener), 140 g (5 oz)
- Cherries, fresh, 110 g (4 oz)
- Damsons, stewed (using artificial sweetener), 110 g (4 oz)
- Dates, fresh, 4
- Grapefruit, pink, half an average fruit
- Grapes, 100 g (3 1/2 oz)
- Greengages, 5 whole
- Mandarins, 2 whole
- Nectarine, 1
- Orange, 1
- Peach, 1
- Pear, 1
- Pineapple, fresh, 110 g (4 oz)
- Pomegranate, 1
- Satsumas, 2
- Strawberries, 200 g (7 oz)
- Tangerines, 2

Small Fruit

Choose one item from this list whenever 'small fruit' is mentioned within your diet:

- Apricots, fresh, 3 whole
- Clementine, 1
- Dates, fresh, 2
- Figs, fresh, 2
- Gooseberries, dessert, raw, 75 g (3 oz)
- Gooseberries, stewed (using artificial sweetener), 140 g (5 oz)

- Grapefruit, white, half an average fruit
- Grapes, 50 g (2 oz)
- Greengages, 3 whole
- Kiwifruit, 1 whole
- Loganberries, stewed (using artificial sweetener), 110 g (4 oz)
- Mandarin orange, 1
- Melon, 200 g (7 oz) slice
- Pineapple, one ring
- Plums, 2 whole fruit
- Raspberries, 110 g (4 oz)
- Rhubarb, stewed (using artificial sweetener), 175 g (6 oz)
- Satsuma, 1
- Strawberries, 110 g (4 oz)
- Tangerine, 1

UNLIMITEDS

General

These items can be used freely on all diets.

Capers, chillies, coffee, oil-free salad dressings, garlic, garlic purée, ground spices of all kinds, pepper, tea, lemon juice, vinegar, water, mineral water, diet calorie-free soft drinks, herb and fruit teas.

Salads

You can eat the following salad items freely within your diet – as between-meal nibbles, as garnishes for your meals, and as instructed within the menus.

- Alfalfa sprouts
- Bamboo shoots, canned
- Beansprouts
- Cabbage, raw, white or red
- Cabbage, red, pickled
- Cauliflower, raw
- Celery
- Chicory
- Chinese leaves
- Chives
- Courgettes, raw
- Cucumber
- Endive
- Fennel
- Gherkins
- Lettuce, all types and colours
- Mint
- Mushrooms, raw
- Mustard and cress
- Onions, raw
- Parsley
- Pepper, green
- Radicchio
- Radishes
- Spring onions
- Watercress

It's time to begin. Turn to your starting diet, and see what food you'll need to get in for tomorrow!

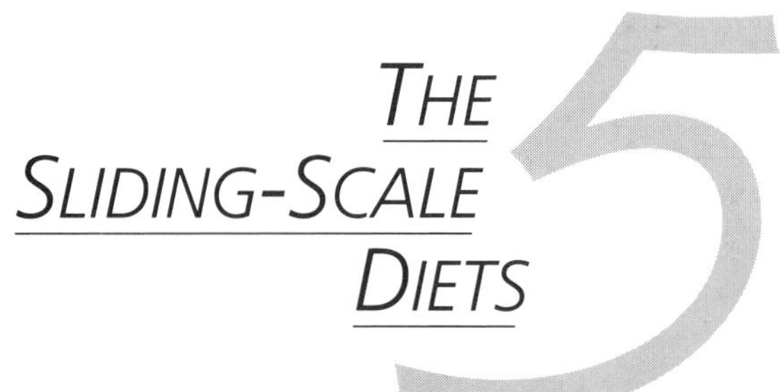

The Sliding-Scale Diets

DIET ONE

IF YOU NEED TO LOSE THREE OR MORE STONE (19 KG +)

Checklist:

- Have your read all the instructions thoroughly?
- Don't forget the extra snacks to which you are entitled (listed on page 28); again, that's three if you're High Met, two if you're Average, and one if you're Low Met.
- Don't forget the foods that are allowed in unlimited quantities each day (listed on page 29).
- When large fruit is mentioned within the diet, choose from the large fruit list on page 28. When small fruit is mentioned, choose from the small fruit list on pages 28–29.
- Your daily skimmed milk allowance on this diet is 250 ml (10 fl oz) per day for use in tea and coffee, unless mentioned otherwise within the diet.
- The set diet beings here. For more flexibility turn to the flexi diet that begins on page 32.
- Remember to stay on this diet until you have only three stone (19 kg) left to lose; then move along to Diet 2, on page 35.
- Remember to fill in all the charts, records and spaces in the boxes provided along the way; they will form your own personal record and will be a real help in your weight-loss campaign.

DAY 1

—— BREAKFAST ——

- 1 small fruit
- 25 g (1 oz) Fruit 'n Fibre or oat bran flakes, with milk from allowance plus 1 medium banana, chopped and mixed in

—— LUNCH ——

- 1 can Weight Watchers Wholesome soup (any variety)
- Sandwich of 2 slices bread with a little low-fat spread, filled with 50 g (2 oz) corned beef *or* tongue, 1 tsp sweet pickle, 1 tomato and plenty of *unlimited* salad items
- 1 small fruit

—— EVENING ——

- 75 g (3 oz) [dry weight] spaghetti, boiled and topped with 1 portion Tomato Sauce (see recipe page 57) with added mushroom (see variation, page 57), plus 2 tsp Parmesan cheese, served with *unlimited* salad items
- 50 g (2 oz) vanilla ice cream *or* 1 125 ml ($4^1/_2$ fl oz) glass dry or medium wine

MY STARTING WEIGHT IS: .... st .... lbs (......... kg)

MY INITIAL TARGET WEIGHT IS: .... st .... lbs (......... kg)

DAY 2

BREAKFAST

• 125 ml (4½ fl oz) low-fat natural yoghurt, with 1 large fruit chopped in, plus 1 tbsp sultanas

LUNCH

• 1 wholemeal pitta bread *or* 2 slices bread, filled with 50 g (2 oz) chopped lean ham, 1 tomato, chopped, *unlimited* chopped salad items of choice, plus seasoning and a pinch of herbs
• 1 large banana

EVENING

• 1 portion Lemon Chicken stir-fry (see recipe, page 66), served with 50 g (2 oz) dried egg noodles, soaked according to manufacturer's instructions

DAY 3

BREAKFAST

• 140 ml (5 fl oz) orange or grapefruit juice
• 2 slices bread with a little low-fat spread and 2 tsp low-sugar jam or marmalade

LUNCH

• 50 g (2 oz) reduced-fat Cheddar-style cheese *or* 40 g (1½ oz) Greek Feta cheese, with a large mixed salad consisting of *unlimited* items, plus tomato, chopped, and 50 g (2 oz) beetroot *or* grated carrot, and 100g (4 oz) reduced-calorie coleslaw
• 1 average wholemeal roll with a little low-fat spread
• 1 small fruit

EVENING

• 1 portion Tandoori Fish Kebabs (see recipe, page 64), served with 65 g (2½ oz) [dry weight] long-grain rice, boiled, plus green salad garnish from *unlimiteds.*

or

• 250 g (9 oz) plain grilled, baked or microwaved white fish fillet, served with 225 g (8 oz) boiled *or* baked potatoes and an average serving (125 g [4½ oz]) broccoli *or* French beans

DAY 4

BREAKFAST

• 140 ml (5 fl oz) orange juice
• 40 g (1½ oz) muesli *or* 2 Weetabix, with milk from allowance

LUNCH

• 1 portion Potato *or* Pea Soup (see recipe and variation, page 58) *or* 425 g (14 oz) can lentil soup
• 65 g (2½ oz) slice French bread with a little low fat spread
• 1 large fruit

EVENING

• 1 portion Cheesy Vegetable Bake (see recipe, page 62) served with a large mixed salad of *unlimited* items

or

• 275 g (10 oz) baked potato, served with 375 g (13 oz) can ratatouille, heated, plus *either* 1 medium-sized egg, poached, *or* 25 g (1 oz) reduced-fat Cheddar cheese, grated

DAY 5

BREAKFAST

• 1 large fruit
• 1 low-calorie diet fruit yoghurt
• 1 slice bread with a little low-fat spread and 1 tsp low-sugar jam or marmalade

LUNCH

• 2 slices bread with a little low-fat spread, filled with 1 medium-sized hard-boiled egg, plenty of *unlimited* salad items, plus 1 tomato and 1 tsp reduced-calorie mayonnaise
• 1 large banana

EVENING

• 1 portion Prawn and Mushroom Risotto (see recipe, page 59) topped with 1 tbsp Parmesan cheese
• 50 g (2 oz) ice cream *or* 1 glass wine

DAY 6

BREAKFAST

• 140 ml (5 fl oz) orange juice
• 1 slice bread, toasted, with a little low-fat spread and topped with 175 g (6 oz) grilled tomatoes *or* with 1 large fruit

LUNCH

• 1 wholemeal pitta bread, warmed, and served with 50 g (2 oz) hummus, plus salad of 50 g (2 oz) canned and drained kidney beans and chopped *unlimited* salad items
• 1 large fruit

EVENING

• 1 portion Chilli Peppers (see recipe, page 68) served with 275 g (10 oz) baked potato

or

• 1 portion Savoury Minced Beef (see recipe, page 68), served with *unlimited* salad items and 225 g (8 oz) baked potato

DAY 7

BREAKFAST

• 140 ml (5 fl oz) orange juice
• 1 medium-sized boiled egg
• 1 slice bread with a little low-fat spread

LUNCH

• Fruity Prawn Salad: mix 75 g (3 oz) peeled prawns with 50 g (2 oz) halved grapes *or* chunks of melon and 1 level tbsp reduced-calorie Thousand Island dressing. Serve on bed of shredded lettuce
• 1 slice bread with a little low-fat spread
• 1 French-style fruit yoghurt and 1 large fruit

EVENING

• 6 mini vegetable burgers (ready-made or from dry mix), served with 1 portion Tomato Sauce (see recipe, page 57), 50 g (2 oz) dried egg noodles *or* pasta (cooked according to manufacturer's instructions) and topped with 1 tbsp Parmesan cheese; green salad from *unlimiteds*

If you need to lose more weight to get down to the 'three stone (19 kg) to go' target, continue on Diet 1 until you reach that level. Or, you have the option of moving to the Flexi diet. If you are now at the 'three stone (19 kg) to go' target, move to Diet 2.

DIET ONE

FLEXIDIET

Many people prefer a set diet when they are slimming; however, your lifestyle – or perhaps your food preferences – may mean that you prefer to choose your own daily menus. In this case, every day choose a breakfast, a lunch and an evening meal from the following lists. The total calorie content of the meals will be approximately the same as the set diet. Extra snacks, unlimiteds and fruits remain unchanged.

BREAKFASTS
(approximately 200 calories each)

Cold

• 40 g ($1^1/_2$ oz) muesli, with milk from allowance; 140 ml (5 fl oz) orange juice
• 125 ml ($4^1/_2$ fl oz) low-fat natural yoghurt mixed with 1 chopped apple and 1 tbsp sultanas or raisins
• 2 slices bread with a little low-fat spread and 1 tsp reduced-sugar jam or marmalade
• 25 g (1 oz) oat bran flakes, with milk from allowance, plus 1 small banana chopped in; 1 small fruit
• 1 diet fruit yoghurt; 1 large fruit; 1 slice bread with a little low-fat spread and 1 tsp low-sugar jam or marmalade
• 25 g (1 oz) bran flakes, with milk from allowance; 1 small fruit; 1 slice bread with a little low-fat spread and 1 tsp pure fruit spread or yeast extract spread

Hot

• 1 slice toast with a little low-fat spread, topped with 3 halved and grilled tomatoes; 140 ml (5 fl oz) orange juice

• 1 slice toast with a little low-fat spread topped with 150 g (5½ oz) baked beans in tomato sauce
• 1 medium-sized egg, boiled or poached; 1 slice bread with a little low-fat spread; 1 small fruit
• 1 average bowl of porridge made half and half with water and skimmed milk; 1 tsp runny honey; 1 large fruit

—— LUNCHES ——

(approximately 400 calories each)

Hot

• 1 portion Potato Soup (see recipe, page 58); 1 wholemeal bap with a little low-fat spread; 1 large fruit
• 213 g (7½ oz) can wholewheat spaghetti in tomato sauce, served on 1 slice toast with a little low-fat spread; 1 large banana
• 175 g (6oz) sliced mushrooms, stir-fried in 1 tsp oil and a little vegetable stock, and served on 2 slices toast; 1 large banana
• 425 g (15oz) can lentil soup; 65 g (2½ oz) slice French bread with a little low-fat spread; 1 small fruit
• 1 warm wholemeal pitta bread filled with 1 portion Chilli Con Carne (see recipe, page 69); *unlimited* salad items plus 1 tomato *or* small fruit
• 2 slices toast with a little low-fat spread, topped with 225 g (8 oz) can baked beans in tomato sauce; 1 small fruit
• 250 g (9 oz) baked potato topped with 100 g (3½ oz) can tuna in tomato sauce; *unlimited* salad items; 1 large fruit
• 250 g (9 oz) baked potato topped with 140 g (5 oz) baked beans in tomato sauce and 25 g (1 oz) grated reduced-fat Cheddar cheese; *unlimited* salad items

Cold (Salads)

• 50 g (2 oz) [dry weight] pasta shapes, boiled and mixed with 50 g (2 oz) cooked chopped chicken, 1 small apple, chopped, 50 g (2 oz) red pepper, chopped, and 50 g (2 oz) sliced mushrooms, all tossed in an oil-free dressing; 1 medium banana
• 50 g (2 oz) [dry weight] long-grain rice, boiled and mixed with 100 g (3½ oz) can tuna in brine, drained and flaked, 25 g (1 oz) cooked peas, 1 stick celery, chopped, 25 g (1 oz) sliced mushrooms, and 25 g (1 oz) sweetcorn, all tossed in an oil-free dressing; 1 small fruit
• 25 g (1 oz) [dry weight] pasta shells, boiled and mixed with 50g (2 oz) reduced-fat Cheddar cheese, chopped, 1 tbsp sultanas, 1 small apple, chopped, and 1 stick celery, all tossed in an oil-free dressing; 1 medium banana

Cold (Packed Lunches)

• 1 large wholemeal bap with a little low-fat spread, filled with 50 g (2 oz) corned beef, 1 tsp sweet pickle and *unlimited* salad items; 1 tomato; 1 large banana
• 2 slices bread with a little low-fat spread, filled with 75 g (3 oz) peeled prawns, tossed in 2 tsp reduced-calorie mayonnaise or salad cream; *unlimited* green salad items; 1 diet fruit yoghurt; 1 small fruit
• 1 sachet instant low-calorie soup of choice; sandwich of 2 slices bread, with a little low-fat spread, filled with 50 g (2 oz) lean ham, French mustard and sliced tomato and spring onions; 1 large banana
• Sandwich of 2 slices bread with a little low-fat spread, filled with 40 g (1½ oz) reduced-fat Cheddar cheese and sliced tomato, plus *unlimited* salad items; 1 diet fruit yoghurt; 1 large fruit
• 3 rye crispbreads with a little low-fat spread; 1 medium-sized hard-boiled egg; 100 g (3½ oz) tub low-fat cottage cheese; *unlimited* salad items; 1 large banana
• Sandwich of 2 slices bread with a little low-fat spread, filled with 50 g (2 oz) lean cooked chicken and *unlimited* salad items; 1 sachet instant low-calorie soup of choice; 1 large fruit; 1 diet fruit yoghurt

—— EVENING MEALS ——

(approximately 500 calories each)

Quick and Easy

• 110 g (4 oz) lean roast beef, leg of lamb or pork (no fat); 225 g (8 oz) baked potato; 100 g (3½ oz) peas; 1 large serving carrots; a little gravy made from stock cube (no added fat); 1 small fruit
• 110 g (4 oz) roast chicken (no skin); 2 average-sized roast potatoes, 1 large serving spring greens;

50 g (2 oz) peas; a little gravy made from stock (no fat)

- 75 g (3 oz) lamb's liver, thinly sliced and dry-fried in a non-stick pan, or well grilled with 1 slice lean back bacon; 200 g (7 oz) instant mashed potato; 110 g (4 oz) broccoli; thin gravy made from stock cube; a little French mustard
- 225 g (8 oz) fillet or steak of white fish, baked or grilled; 225 g (8 oz) baked or boiled potato; 110 g (4 oz) carrots
- 110 g (4 oz) pork tenderloin, grilled; 1 tbsp apple sauce; 175 g (6 oz) new potatoes; 150 g ($5^1/_2$ oz) broccoli or mangetout
- 75 g (3 oz) [dry weight] long pasta of choice (i.e., spaghetti or tagliatelle), boiled and topped with half a 475 g (16 oz) jar Napoletana sauce with vegetables; 1 tbsp Parmesan cheese; *unlimited* salad items; 1 small fruit
- 250 g (9 oz) frozen stir-fry rice, peas and mushrooms (cooked according to manufacturer's instructions) with addition of *either* 1 raw egg (stirred until cooked) *or* 50 g (2 oz) lean cooked chicken or ham, chopped; *unlimited* salad items; 1 large banana
- 150 g ($5^1/_2$ oz) chicken portion, grilled and served with 225 g (8 oz) can ready-cooked brown rice, and 75 g (3 oz) sweetcorn; 1 large fruit

Recipe dishes

- 1 portion Fish Moussaka (see recipe, page 63); 100 g ($3^1/_2$ oz) green beans; 1 large fruit
- 1 portion Lemon Chicken Stir-fry (see recipe, page 66) with 50 g (2 oz) [dry weight] egg noodles, soaked according to manufacturer's instructions)
- 1 portion Chilli Peppers (see recipe, page 68); 250 g (9 oz) baked potato
- 75 g (3 oz) [dry weight] spaghetti, boiled and topped with 1 portion Bolognese Sauce (see recipe, page 58)
- 1 portion Tomato and Ham Tagliatelle (see recipe, page 59); *unlimited* salad items; 1 small fruit
- 1 portion Cod Creole (see recipe, page 64); 1 large fruit
- 1 portion Cheesy Chicken and Pasta (see recipe, page 60); 1 large fruit
- 1 Lamb Burger (see recipe, page 69); 225 g (8 oz) boiled potato; 100 g ($3^1/_2$ oz) broad beans or peas
- 1 portion Haddock and Spinach Layer (see recipe, page 65); 175 g (6 oz) mashed or boiled potato; 1 small fruit
- 1 portion Tuna and Broccoli Bake (see recipe, page 64); 150 g ($5^1/_2$ oz) boiled potatoes

Vegetarian Meals

- 1 portion Vegetable Curry (see recipe, page 63) with 140 g (5 oz) [cooked weight] rice
- Vegetarian Feasts Spinach and Walnut Lasagne; *unlimited* salad items; 1 large banana
- Healthy Options Vegetable Tandoori Curry; mini wholemeal pitta bread
- 1 portion Chow Mein (see recipe, page 59); 1 large fruit
- 1 portion Savoury Lentil Crumble (see recipe, page 62); *unlimited* salad items; 1 small fruit
- 1 portion Cheesy Vegetable Bake (see recipe, page 62); 1 large fruit
- 3 Vegetarian sausages (ready-made, or prepared from a mix); 140 g (5 oz) baked beans; 175 g (6 oz) instant mashed potato; 1 large fruit

Ready-made Meals

NB: Try to limit ready-made meals to a maximum of two a week.

- $^1/_2$ x McCain Ham and Mushroom Deep Pan Pizza; *unlimited* salad items; 1 large fruit
- Healthy Options Spaghetti Bolognese; *unlimited* salad items; 1 large banana
- 250 g (9 oz) Dolmio Chilled Beef and Tomato Ravioli; *unlimited* salad items
- Birds Eye Menu Master Beef Curry and Rice; green salad from *unlimiteds*; 1 large banana
- Birds Eye Menu Master Chinese Chicken and Rice; *unlimited* salad items plus 1 tomato; 1 large fruit

End of Diet 1:

Today I weigh .... st .... lbs (......... kg)

I have lost a total of .... lbs (......... kg)

since the beginning of the diet.

DIET TWO

IIF YOU NEED TO LOSE BETWEEN TWO AND THREE STONE (12.7 –19 KG)

Checklist:

- Have you thoroughly read all the instructions on pages 25–29?
- Don't forget the extra snacks to which you are entitled (listed on page 28); again, three if you're High Met, two if you're Average, one if you're Low Met.
- Don't forget your daily *unlimiteds* (listed on page 29); you can eat any of these foods freely.
- Large fruit and small fruit lists appear on pages 28–29.
- Your daily skimmed milk allowance on this diet is 250 ml (9 fl oz) a day for use in tea and coffee, unless mentioned otherwise within the diet.
- The set diet begins here. For more flexibility turn to the flexi diet that begins on page 37.
- Remember to stay on this diet until you have only two stone (12.7 kg) left to lose; then move along to Diet 3, on page 40.
- Remember to fill in all the charts, records and spaces in the boxes provided along the way; they will form your own personal record and will be a real help in your weight-loss campaign.

MY STARTING WEIGHT IS:

.... st .... lbs (......... kg)

MY INITIAL TARGET WEIGHT IS:

.... st .... lbs (......... kg)

- Never skip a meal. Eat everything you are allowed. If you don't eat something you are allowed, save it for later in the day.
- Try to space your meals evenly throughout the day and leave at least two hours between eating and going to bed.
- Eat slowly and chew your food well. Taking time to enjoy your food will make you feel fuller.
- Drink as much water as you like, particularly with meals. This will help fill you up as well as aiding your digestion.

DAY 1

BREAKFAST

- 40 g (1½ oz) muesli, with milk from allowance, plus 1 large fruit chopped in

LUNCH

- 75 g (3 oz) slice French bread with a little low-fat spread, with 100 g (3½oz) low-calorie coleslaw and 50 g (2oz) smoked turkey or ham, plus *unlimited* salad items

EVENING

- 1 portion Chilli Con Carne (see recipe, page 69), served with 50 g (2 oz) [dry weight] long-grain rice, boiled (cook extra rice for tomorrow's lunch)

DAY 2

BREAKFAST

- 110 ml (4 fl oz) orange juice
- 125 ml (4½ fl oz) low-fat natural yoghurt, with 15 g (½ oz) bran flakes and half an apple chopped in

LUNCH

- 1 portion Rice Salad with Tuna (see recipe, page 60)
- 1 large banana

or

- Sandwich of 2 slices bread with a little low-fat spread, filled with 100 g (3½ oz) can tuna in brine, drained and mashed, plus *unlimited* salad items and 1 tomato, sliced
- 1 large banana

EVENING

- 1 portion Caribbean Chicken (see recipe, page 67), served with 50 g (2 oz) [dry weight] long-grain rice, boiled, and green salad from *unlimited* items

or

- 150 g (5½ oz) grilled chicken portion with rice and green salad from *unlimited* items
- 1 small fruit

DAY 3

BREAKFAST

• 1 slice bread, toasted, topped with 1 medium banana mashed with a little lemon juice and cinnamon
• 1 small fruit

LUNCH

• 3 rye crispbreads spread with 15 g (1/2 oz) peanut butter, and topped with slices of apple and celery
• 1 large fruit

EVENING

• 1 portion Meat-free Bolognese (see variation to Bolognese recipe, page 58), served with 50 g (2 oz) [dry weight] pasta of choice, boiled, plus *unlimited* salad items

or

• 1 Lean Quarterpounder beefburger in 1 large wholemeal bap, plus *unlimited* salad items

DAY 4

BREAKFAST

• 25 g (1 oz) Special K or bran flakes, with 140 ml (5 fl oz) skimmed milk, extra to allowance, and 1 large fruit chopped in

LUNCH

• 75 g (3 oz) French bread, 40 g (1 1/2 oz) reduced-fat Cheddar-style cheese, 2 tsp sweet pickle, a little low-fat spread, plus a large salad of *unlimited* items

EVENING

• 2 Tuna Fish Cakes (see recipe, page 64), served with 110 g (4 oz) peas and a large portion broccoli
• 50 g (2 oz) ice cream or 1 glass dry wine

or

• 140 g (5 oz) smoked haddock fillet, grilled, baked or poached, served with 175 g (6oz) boiled potatoes, 7 g (1/4 oz) low-fat spread, broccoli and peas as above
• 1 small fruit

DAY 5

BREAKFAST

• 125 ml (4 1/2 fl oz) low-fat natural yoghurt with 1 tsp runny honey plus 1 large fruit chopped in, and 15 g (1/2 oz) bran flakes or Special K sprinkled on top

LUNCH

• Sandwich of 2 slices bread with a little low-fat spread, filled with 50 g (2 oz) lean ham and *unlimited* salad items, plus 1 tomato
• 1 large banana

EVENING

• 1 portion Vegetable Curry (see recipe, page 63), served with 25 g (1oz) [dry weight] long-grain rice, boiled

DAY 6

BREAKFAST

• 1 1/2 slices bread with a little low-fat spread, topped with 2 tsp reduced-sugar jam or marmalade
• 1 large fruit

LUNCH

• 3 rye crispbreads with tuna pâté: mash 100 g (3 1/2 oz) can tuna in brine, drained, with 75 g (3 oz) low-fat soft cheese and seasoning, plus *unlimited* salad items
• 1 large fruit

EVENING

• 1 portion Nutty Chicken with Beansprouts (see recipe, page 68), served with 50 g (2oz) dried egg noodles (cooked according to manufacturer's instructions) or with 50 g (2oz) [dry weight] rice, boiled

or

• 110 g (4 oz) roast chicken (no skin), served with 225 g (8oz) baked potato, 110 g (4 oz) carrots and 50 g (2 oz) sweetcorn, plus a little thin gravy made from stock cube

DAY 7

—— BREAKFAST ——

- 140 ml (5 fl oz) orange juice
- 1 medium-sized egg, boiled
- 1 slice bread with a little low-fat spread

—— LUNCH ——

- 1 wholemeal pitta bread, served with 75 g (3 oz) hummus and a sliced tomato and onion side salad

—— EVENING ——

- 1 portion Cod Creole (see recipe, page 64)

or

- 1 frozen cod steak in wholemeal crumbs, baked or grilled, served with 225 g (8oz) mashed potato and 50 g (2 oz) peas

If you need to lose more weight to get down to the 'two stone (12.7 kg) to go' target, continue on Diet 2 until you reach that level. Or, you have the option of moving to the flexi diet. If you are now at the 'two stone (12.7 kg) to go' target, move to Diet 3.

DIET TWO

FLEXIDIET

Many people prefer a set diet when they are slimming; however, your lifestyle – or perhaps your food preferences – may mean that you prefer to choose your own daily menus. In this case, every day choose a breakfast, a lunch and an evening meal from the following lists. The total calorie content of the meals will be approximately the same as the set diet. Extra snacks, unlimiteds and fruits remain unchanged.

—— BREAKFAST ——

(approximately 200 calories each)

Cold

- 40 g (1½ oz) muesli, with milk from allowance; 1 large fruit
- 25 g (1 oz) Special K, with milk from allowance; 1 large banana
- 25 g (1 oz) bran flakes, with 1 large fruit and 1 tbsp dried fruit of choice; milk from allowance
- 125 ml (4½ oz) low-fat natural yoghurt with 1 tsp runny honey; 1 banana
- 2 slices bread with a little low-fat spread and 2 tsp low-sugar jam or marmalade
- 25 g (1 oz) Fruit 'n Fibre, with milk from allowance; 1 slice bread with a little low-fat spread and 1 tsp low-sugar jam or marmalade

Hot

- 1 slice toast with a little low-fat spread, topped with 1 large banana mashed with a little lemon juice and cinnamon
- 1 medium-sized egg, boiled or poached, with 1 slice toast and a little low-fat spread; 1 small fruit
- 1 slice toast with a little low fat spread, topped with 150 g (5½ oz) baked beans in tomato sauce
- 1 average bowl porridge, made half and half with water and skimmed milk; 1 level tsp brown sugar; 1 large fruit
- 175 g (6 oz) mushrooms baked or microwaved in their own juices and seasoning, on 2 slices toast with a little low fat spread

— LUNCHES —
(approximately 350 calories each)

Hot

• 1 large wholemeal bap, halved and toasted, topped with 50 g (2 oz) reduced-fat Cheddar cheese, sliced, and grilled until bubbling; 1 tomato; 1 large fruit
• 425 g (15oz) can pea and ham soup; 50 g (2 oz) slice wholemeal French bread *or* 1 *petit pain* with a little low-fat spread; 1 small fruit
• 1 warm wholemeal pitta bread filled with 1 portion Bolognese Sauce (see recipe, page 58)
• 225 g (8 oz) baked potato, topped with 75 g (3 oz) baked beans and 25 g (1 oz) grated reduced-fat Cheddar cheese; *unlimited* salad items
• 1 portion Potato *or* Pea soup (see recipes, page 58); 1 slice bread with a little low-fat spread; 1 large banana

Cold (Salads)

• 1 portion Rice Salad with Tuna (see recipe, page 60); 1 large banana
• 1 medium-sized hard-boiled egg, sliced and mixed with 75 g (3 oz) peeled prawns and 2 tsp reduced-calorie mayonnaise, served on a bed of *unlimited* green salad items; 2 slices bread with a little low-fat spread
• Salad Nicoise: combine 1 small lettuce heart, quartered, with shredded lettuce leaves, $3^1/_2$ oz (100 g) can tuna in brine, drained, 1 medium-sized hard-boiled egg, chopped, 1 tomato, quartered, 4 stoned black olives, 25 g (1 oz) cooked French beans; toss all in an oil-free salad dressing; 1 average wholemeal roll with a little low-fat spread

Cold (Packed Lunches)

• Sandwich of 2 slices bread with a little low-fat spread, filled with 100 g ($3^1/_2$ oz) cottage cheese and *unlimited* salad items, plus 1 tomato; 1 diet fruit yoghurt; 1 large fruit
• Sandwich of 2 slices bread with a little low-fat spread, filled with 50 g (2 oz) lean roast beef and horseradish sauce, plus lettuce; 1 sachet instant low-calorie soup of choice; 1 large fruit
• Boots Shapers Chicken and Chinese Leaf sandwich; 1 large fruit; 1 medium banana
• Sandwich of 2 slices bread with a little low-fat spread, filled with medium-sized hard-boiled egg and salad; 1 diet fruit yoghurt; 1 large fruit
• 50 g (2 oz) reduced-fat Cheddar cheese; 3 rye crispbreads; 1 tomato; 1 large fruit; 1 muesli bar

— EVENING MEALS —
(approximately 450 calories each)

Quick and Easy

• 110 g (4oz) gammon rasher, well grilled; 225 g (8 oz) boiled potatoes; 50 g (2 oz) sweetcorn
• 1 skinned chicken breast fillet, sprinkled with barbecue seasoning and grilled; 1 wholemeal bap with a little low-fat spread; *unlimited* salad items
• Omelette made from 2 medium-sized eggs, beaten with a little water and seasoning, with 40 g ($1^1/_2$ oz) lean ham, chopped, and cooked in 7 g ($^1/_4$ oz) low-fat spread in a non-stick pan; 1 wholemeal roll with a little low-fat spread; *unlimited* salad items, plus 1 tomato
• 225 g (8 oz) baked potato topped with 100 g ($3^1/_2$ oz) can tuna in brine, drained and flaked, mixed with 50 g (2oz) sweetcorn and 2 tbsp low-fat natural fromage frais; 1 large fruit
• 200 g (7 oz) grilled trout; 140 g (5oz) mashed potato; 100 g ($3^1/_2$ oz) peas; 1 small fruit
• 110 g (4 oz) lean roast beef; 140 g (5 oz) new potatoes; 140 g (5 oz) cabbage; 100 g ($3^1/_2$ oz) carrots; a little thin gravy made from stock cube
• 110 g (4 oz) fillet pork, cubed, coated with 1 tbsp Hoi Sin sauce and threaded on kebab stick, grilled until tender; 50 g (2 oz) [dry weight] long-grain rice, boiled; *unlimited* green salad items
• Stir-fry of 110 g (4 oz) chicken meat, sliced, and a selection of finely-sliced vegetables of choice with 80 g (3 oz) ready-made sweet and sour sauce; 50 g (2 oz) [dry weight] long-grain rice, boiled; *unlimited* green salad items

Recipe Dishes

• 1 portion Chilli Con Carne (see recipe, page 69); 50 g (2 oz) [dry weight] long-grain rice, boiled, *or* 225 g (8 oz) baked potato; 1 large fruit

TEN NON-FATTENING ALTERNATIVES TO FORBIDDEN FOODS

- Ring up a friend.
- Write a letter.
- Begin that best-selling novel.
- Tidy your dresser/wardrobe.
- See what clothes you can alter/adapt for when you are slim.
- Read the holiday brochures.
- Pick some flowers from the garden and make an arrangement.
- Make a plan for the next twelve months. Divide it into Work, Home/Family, Friends and Leisure, and write down all the short-term and long-term things you would like to achieve, from the easy to the near impossible! Over the days ahead, work out strategies.
- Start a file of low-fat high-carbohydrate recipes to try when you are on your maintenance plan.
- Write a list of all the things you'd like for your birthday or Christmas.

• 1 portion Caribbean Chicken (see recipe, page 67); 50 g (2 oz) [dry weight] long-grain rice, boiled; *unlimited* salad items
• 1 portion Pork and Pineapple Stir-Fry (see recipe, page 69); 40 g (1½ oz) [dry weight] egg noodles, soaked according to manufacturer's instructions
• 1 portion Nutty Chicken with Beansprouts (see recipe, page 68); 40 g (1½ oz) [dry weight] long-grain rice, boiled
• 1 portion Sweet and Sour Stir-Fry (see recipe, page 65); 50 g (2 oz) [dry weight] egg noodles, soaked according to manufacturer's instructions
• 1 portion Chilli Chicken with Aromatic Rice (see recipe, page 66); 1 large fruit
• 1 portion Potato and Ham Stir-Fry (see recipe, page 62); *unlimited* salad items and 1 tomato; 1 large banana

Vegetarian Meals

• 4 Birds Eye Crispy Vegetable Fingers, grilled; 175 g (6 oz) instant mashed potato; 140 g (5 oz) baked beans; 1 large fruit
• 1 portion Meat-free Bolognese (recipe variation; see page 58); 50 g (2 oz) [dry weight] spaghetti, boiled; 1 small fruit or *unlimited* salad items and 1 tomato
• 1 portion Vegetable Curry (see recipe, page 63); 25 g (1oz) [dry weight] long-grain rice, boiled
• 1 portion Nut Pilaff (see recipe, page 60); *unlimited* salad items; 1 small fruit
• 1 portion Red Pepper Pasta (vegetarian option; see recipe, page 61); *unlimited* salad items; 1 small fruit
• Mushroom omelette made with 2 medium-sized eggs and 75 g (3oz) sliced button mushrooms; 1 wholemeal bap with a little low-fat spread; *unlimited* salad items; 1 medium banana
• 275 g (10 oz) baked potato with easy cheese sauce: melt down 150 g (6 oz) pot low-fat soft cheese, and spoon over potato; *unlimited* salad items

Ready-made Meals

NB: Try to limit ready-made meals to a maximum of two a week.

• Healthy Options Seafood Tagliatelle; *unlimited* salad items; 1 small fruit
• Birds Eye Roast Turkey Platter; 1 large fruit
• Findus Cannelloni; 1 small fruit *or unlimited* salad items, plus 1 tomato

End of Diet 2:

Today I weigh .... st .... lbs (......... kg)

I have lost a total of .... lbs (......... kg) since the beginning of the diet.

DIET THREE

IF YOU NEED TO LOSE BETWEEN ONE AND TWO STONE (6.4–12.7 KG)

Checklist:

- Have you thoroughly read all the instructions on pages 25–29?
- Don't forget the extra snacks to which you are entitled (listed on page 28); again, that's three if you're High Met, two if you're Average, and one if you're Low Met.
- Don't forget the foods that are allowed in unlimited quantities each day (listed on page 29).
- Large fruit and small fruit lists appear on pages 28–29.
- Your daily skimmed milk allowance on this diet is 125 ml (4½ fl oz) per day for use in tea and coffee, unless mentioned otherwise within the diet.
- The set diet beings here. For more flexibility turn to the flexi diet that begins on page 42.
- Remember to stay on this diet until you have only one stone (6.4 kg) left to lose; then move along to Diet 4, on page 45.
- Remember to fill in all the charts, records and spaces in the boxes provided along the way; they will form your own personal record and will be a real help in your weight-loss campaign.

MY STARTING WEIGHT IS:

.... st .... lbs (......... kg)

MY INITIAL TARGET WEIGHT IS:

.... st .... lbs (......... kg)

Always check through each days's menu to make sure all the foods it contains are ones that you enjoy. If there is something on a particular day's menu that is not to your liking, then switch to the flexi diet for the whole of that day. Keep a note of your favourite recipes so that you can try them again when you move on to the maintenance diet. Remember to make full use of your unlimiteds. These will help fill you up and make your meal look more appetising.

DAY 1

BREAKFAST

- 1 small fruit
- 25 g (1 oz) bran flakes or Fruit 'n Fibre, with 110 ml (4 fl oz) skimmed milk, extra to allowance

LUNCH

- 425 g (15 oz) can lentil soup
- 1 average wholemeal roll with a little low-fat spread
- 1 small fruit

or

- 1 large wholemeal bap with a little low-fat spread, filled with 50 g (2 oz) lean turkey or chicken and *unlimited* salad items
- 1 small fruit

EVENING

- Fish parcel: place a 250 g (9 oz) fillet of white fish on a large piece of foil; add some slivers of celery and carrot, lemon juice, seasoning and fresh herbs (e.g., chopped chives) to taste; seal and bake or microwave until fish is tender Serve with 250 g (9 oz) new or baked potatoes and 125 g (4½ oz) broccoli or green beans

DAY 2

BREAKFAST

125 ml (4½ fl oz) low-fat natural yogurt, with 2 tsp sultanas or raisins, and 1 chopped apple

LUNCH

- Sandwich of 2 slices bread with a little low-fat spread, filled with 1 medium-sized hard-boiled egg, *unlimited* salad items, plus 1 tomato
- 1 large banana

EVENING

- 1 portion Red Pepper Pasta (see recipe, page 61), served with green salad from *unlimited* items
- 1 small fruit

DAY 3

— BREAKFAST —

- 1 slice bread with a little low-fat spread, and 1 heaped tsp low-sugar jam or marmalade
- 1 large fruit

or

- $1^{1}/_{2}$ slices bread, toasted, and topped with 3 tomatoes, halved and grilled

— LUNCH —

- 4 tbsp ready-made 3-bean salad; plus 1 average wholemeal roll with a little low-fat spread and a large mixed salad of *unlimited* items, plus tomato or beetroot

— EVENING —

- 1 portion Thai Chicken (see recipe, page 67), served with 40 g ($1^{1}/_{2}$ oz) dried egg noodles, soaked according to manufacturer's instructions

or

- 110 g (4 oz) lean chicken, sliced, plus finely sliced vegetables of choice, stir-fried with 3 oz (80 g) ready-made sweet and sour sauce, plus 50 g (2 oz) [dry weight] egg noodles, soaked according to manufacturer's instructions

AVOID TEMPTATION!

When you are starting your weight-loss campaign, it will help if you clear out the larder and refrigerator before you begin.

- Go through the fridge and give anything you don't need to friends, or throw it away.
- Eat before you go shopping – that way you won't be tempted to buy items you don't need and which you can't resist because you feel hungry.
- Think before you buy. Do you really need that packet of biscuits?
- Always check the labels on items before you purchase them. If low-fat or reduced-sugar varieties are avalable, choose them in place of those which contain more calories.

DAY 4

— BREAKFAST —

- 25 g (1 oz) Special K or Fruit 'n Fibre, with 125 ml ($4^{1}/_{2}$ fl oz) skimmed milk, extra to allowance

— LUNCH —

- 3 rye crispbreads with a little low-fat spread, topped with 75 g (3 oz) pink salmon *or* 100 g ($3^{1}/_{2}$ oz) can tuna, plus *unlimited* salad items
- 1 medium banana and 1 diet fruit fromage frais

— EVENING —

- Barbecued rice with black-eye beans: cook half a packet of savoury rice and mushrooms according to manufacturer's instructions; add 1 tbsp barbecue or sweet and sour sauce and contents of $3^{1}/_{2}$ oz (100 g) can black-eye beans; warm through and serve

or

- 250 g (9 oz) baked potato, topped with 1 portion Chilli Con Carne (see recipe, page 69) and serve with a large salad of *unlimited* items

DAY 5

— BREAKFAST —

- 125 ml ($4^{1}/_{2}$ fl oz) low-fat natural yoghurt, mixed with 2 tbsp muesli
- 1 small fruit

— LUNCH —

- 75 g (3 oz) hummus with 1 wholemeal pitta, plus a Mediterranean salad of tomatoes, peppers, onion and halved stoned black olives, tossed in an oil-free dressing

— EVENING —

- 1 portion Speedy Bolognese Sauce (see recipe, page 58) on 50 g (2 oz) [dry weight] pasta of choice, boiled, and sprinkled with 2 tsp Parmesan cheese, served with green salad items from *unlimiteds* list.

DAY 6

— BREAKFAST —

• 1 small fruit
• 1 slice bread with 25 g (1 oz) reduced-fat cheese spread

— LUNCH —

• 225 g (8 oz) can baked beans in tomato sauce, served on 2 slices toast with a little low-fat spread
• 1 small fruit

or

• Sandwich of 2 slices bread with a little low-fat spread, filled with 100 g ($3^1/_2$ oz) can tuna in brine, drained, plus *unlimited* salad items
• 1 large fruit

— EVENING —

• 1 portion Chilli Chicken with Aromatic Rice (see recipe, page 60), served with *unlimited* side salad

or

• 175 g (6 oz) chicken portion, grilled (with skin removed), served with Vegetable Rice, (see recipe, page 60) *or* with 225 g (8 oz) baked potato and a large salad from *unlimited* items

DAY 7

— BREAKFAST —

• 1 small fruit
• 1 medium-sized egg, boiled
• 1 slice bread with a little low-fat spread

— LUNCH —

• 75 g (3 oz) slice French bread with 40 g ($1^1/_2$ oz) reduced-fat Cheddar cheese *or* Brie; 1 tsp sweet pickle; *unlimited* salad items, plus 1 tomato

— EVENING —

• 1 portion Sweet and Sour Stir-fry (see recipe, page 65) served with 50 g (2 oz) [dry weight] long-grain rice, boiled, and green salad garnish from *unlimiteds*

or

• 225 g (8 oz) fillet of monkfish or cod baked, grilled or microwaved, and served with 200 g (7 oz) boiled or baked potato and 150 g ($5^1/_2$ oz) green beans

> If you need to lose more weight to get down to the 'one stone to go' target, continue on Diet 3 until you reach that level. Or, you have the option of moving to the flexi diet. If you are now at the 'one stone to go' target, move to Diet 4.

DIET THREE
FLEXIDIET

Many people prefer a set diet when they are slimming; however, your lifestyle – or perhaps your food preferences – may mean that you prefer to choose your own daily menus. In this case, every day choose a breakfast, a lunch and an evening meal from the following lists. The total calorie content of the meals will be approximately the same as the set diet. Your daily skimmed milk allowance, extra snacks, unlimiteds and fruits remain unchanged.

— BREAKFASTS —
(approximately 150 calories each)

Cold

• 1 small fruit; 25 g (1 oz) Bran Buds or All Bran, with 110 ml (4 fl oz) skimmed milk, extra to allowance
• 125 ml ($4^1/_2$ fl oz) low-fat natural yoghurt mixed with 2 tsp raisins or sultanas and 1 chopped small apple

• 1 slice bread with a little low-fat spread and 1 tsp low-sugar jam or marmalade; 1 small fruit
• 25 g (1 oz) Special K or Fruit 'n Fibre, with 110 ml (4 fl oz) skimmed milk extra to allowance
• 125 ml (4½ fl oz) low-fat natural yoghurt with 15 g (½ oz) muesli and 1 small fruit mixed in
• 15 g (½ oz) Puffed Wheat, with 100 ml (3½ fl oz) skimmed milk extra to allowance; 1 large fruit
• 1 diet fruit yoghurt; 1 large banana

Hot

• 1 slice toast with a little low-fat spread, topped with 75 g (3 oz) baked beans
• 1 slice toast with a little low-fat spread, topped with 1 medium banana mashed with a little lemon juice and cinnamon
• 1 medium-sized egg, boiled or poached; 1 slice toast with a little low-fat spread
• 1 slice toast, topped with 140 g (5 oz) mushrooms, baked or microwaved in foil with lemon juice, seasoning and 7 g (¼ oz) added low-fat spread
• 1 slice toast with a little low-fat spread, topped with 2 tomatoes, halved and grilled

—— LUNCHES ——

(approximately 350 calories each)

Hot

• 213 g (7½ oz) can wholewheat spaghetti in tomato sauce, served on 2 slices toast with a little low-fat spread; 1 large fruit
• 2 medium-sized eggs, scrambled with a little low-fat spread and skimmed milk from your allowance; 2 slices toast with a little low-fat spread
• 1 medium-sized egg, poached, and 1 slice lean back bacon, well grilled; 1 wholemeal roll with a little low fat spread; 1 large fruit
• 225 g (8 oz) baked potato, topped with 140 g (5 oz) baked beans; 1 large fruit
• 225 g (8 oz) can baked beans on 2 slices toast; 1 small fruit

Cold (Salads)

• Chicken coleslaw: mix 110 g (4 oz) shredded white cabbage, 50 g (2 oz) grated carrot, 25 g (1 oz) grated onion, 25 g (1 oz) sultanas and 50 g (2 oz) lean cooked chopped chicken. Stir into this a dressing: 1 tbsp low-fat natural yoghurt mixed with 1 level tbsp reduced-calorie mayonnaise, seasoning and 1 tsp lemon juice; 1 large banana
• Feta salad: crumble 40 g (1½ oz) Greek Feta cheese and mix with 1 beef tomato, chopped, 1 chunk cucumber, chopped, 1 small green pepper, de-seeded and chopped, 5 black olives, stoned, and a little chopped crisp lettuce. Drizzle with oil-free salad dressing; 1 wholemeal roll with a little low-fat spread; 1 large fruit

Cold (Packed Lunches)

• Sandwich of 2 slices bread with a little low-fat spread, filled with 50 g (2 oz) corned beef, 1 sliced tomato and *unlimited* salad items; 1 large fruit or 1 diet fruit yoghurt
• Ploughman's sandwich: fill a 50 g (2 oz) slice French bread with a little low-fat spread, 40 g (1½ oz) reduced-fat Cheddar cheese, 50 g (2 oz) diet coleslaw and *unlimited* salad items
• Sandwich of 2 slices bread with a little low-fat spread, filled with 50 g (2 oz) lean cooked chicken, tossed in 2 tsp low-fat natural yoghurt mixed with 1 tsp reduced-calorie mayonnaise, and pinch curry powder; *unlimited* salad items; 1 medium banana
• Sandwich of 2 slices bread with a little low-fat spread, filled with 50 g (2 oz) lean ham, French mustard, *unlimited* salad items, and 1 sliced tomato; 1 diet fruit yoghurt; 1 small fruit
• 3 rye crispbreads with a little low-fat spread; 40 g (1½ oz) Brie; *unlimited* items; 1 small fruit; 1 diet fromage frais

—— EVENING MEALS ——

(approximately 450 calories each)

Quick and Easy

• Fish parcel: wrap 250 g (9 oz) fish steak or fillet in foil with lemon juice, seasoning and a few very thin strips of carrot and celery, and bake until tender; 225 g (8 oz) new potatoes; 150 g (5½ oz) broccoli or mangetout
• 1 medium-sized poached egg; 2 well-grilled slices lean back bacon; 75 g (3 oz) mushrooms; 1 large

tomato, sliced and grilled; 1 slice bread with a little low-fat spread
• 4 pork spare ribs, Chinese-style, baked; 225 g (8 oz) [cooked weight] long-grain rice, boiled; *unlimited* salad items; 1 small fruit
• 140 g (5 oz) lean chicken meat cut into cubes and skewered, grilled; 2 tbsp ready-made peanut sauce; *unlimited* salad items
• Lean quarterpounder beefburger, grilled; 225 g (8 oz) instant mashed potato; 75 g (3 oz) baked beans in tomato sauce
• 110 g (4 oz) lean roast chicken; 225 g (8 oz) baked potato; large serving cabbage; 110 g (4 oz) carrots; a little thin gravy made from stock cube
• 2 salmon fishcakes, grilled; 225 g (8 oz) instant mashed or boiled potato; 75 g (3 oz) peas
• 140 g (5 oz) fillet steak, grilled; 225 g (8 oz) baked potato; *unlimited* salad items
• 75 g (3 oz) [dry weight] pasta of choice topped with contents of 200 g (7 oz) jar Italian tomato sauce; *unlimited* salad items
• 4 breaded cod fish fingers, grilled; 225 g (8 oz) instant mashed or boiled potato; 75 g (3 oz) peas, sweetcorn or baked beans

Recipe Dishes

• 1 portion Fish Moussaka (see recipe, page 63); 1 small fruit
• 1 portion Thai Chicken (see recipe, page 67) with 40 g ($1^1/_2$ oz) [dry weight] long-grain rice or noodles, boiled
• 1 portion Lemon Chicken Stir-Fry (see recipe, page 66) with 40 g ($1^1/_2$ oz) [dry weight] pasta shells, boiled
• 1 portion Savoury Minced Beef (see recipe, page 68) topped with 200 g (7 oz) mashed potato and browned under grill; 140 g (5 oz) green beans
• 1 portion Prawn and Mushroom Risotto (see recipe, page 59); 1 medium banana
• 1 portion Tuna and Broccoli Bake (see recipe, page 64); 110 g (4 oz) boiled potato
• 1 portion Tomato and Ham Tagliatelle (see recipe, page 59); *unlimited* green salad items
• 1 portion Red Pepper Pasta (see recipe, page 61); 1 large fruit

Vegetarian Meals

• 1 portion Chow Mein, (see recipe, page 59); 1 small fruit
• 225 g (8 oz) baked potato with 1 portion meat-free Bolognese sauce (see recipe variation, page 58); *unlimited* salad items
• 1 vegetable burger, grilled; 50 g (2 oz) [dry weight] noodles, soaked according to manufacturer's instructions, topped with 1 portion Tomato Sauce (see recipe, page 57); 1 large fruit
• Vegetarian Feasts Tasty Lentil Bake; *unlimited* salad items; 1 large banana
• 1 portion Cheesy Vegetable Bake (see recipe, page 62)
• RealEat Vege Lasagne; *unlimited* salad items; 1 large fruit

Ready-made Meals

NB: Try to limit ready-made meals to a maximum of two a week.

• Birds Eye Menu Master Beef Curry with Rice; 1 large fruit
• Findus Lasagne; 1 small fruit
• Healthy Options Chicken Chasseur with Rice; *unlimited* green salad items
• Individual Shepherd's/Cottage pie (ready-made; maximum 400 calories); 1 large fruit

End of Diet 3:

Today I weigh .... st .... lbs (......... kg)

I have lost a total of .... lbs (......... kg) since the beginning of the diet.

DIET FOUR

IF YOU NEED TO LOSE BETWEEN A HALF AND ONE STONE (3.2–6.4 KG)

Checklist:

- Have your thoroughly read all the instructions (on pages 25–29)?
- Don't forget the extra snacks to which you are entitled (listed on page 28); again, that's three if you're High Met, two if you're Average, and one if you're Low Met.
- Don't forget the foods that are allowed in unlimited quantities each day (listed on page 29).
- Large fruit and small fruit lists appear on pages 28–29.
- Your daily skimmed milk allowance on this diet is 125 ml (4½ fl oz) per day for use in tea and coffee, unless mentioned otherwise within the diet.
- The set diet beings here. For more flexibility turn to the flexi diet that begins on page 47.
- Remember to stay on this diet until you have only half a stone (3.2 kg) left to lose; then move along to Diet 5, on page 49.
- Remember to fill in all the charts, records and spaces in the boxes provided along the way; they will form your own personal record and will be a real help in your weight-loss campaign.

MY STARTING WEIGHT IS:

.... st .... lbs (......... kg)

MY INITIAL TARGET WEIGHT IS:

.... st .... lbs (......... kg)

Everyone has those difficult days when it seems almost impossible to stick to the diet. Don't give up. If you have an urge to eat a bar of chocolate or a slice of cake, try eating one of the snacks from the lists on page 28 instead to limit the potential damage. If you do end up eating more than you should, don't use this as an excuse to abandon the diet. Just get straight back to the diet the following day. If you've had a serious lapse, try the Speed Plus Plan on pages 55–56 for a day or two.

DAY 1

— BREAKFAST —

- 15 g (½ oz) Puffed Wheat, with 100 ml (3½ fl oz) skimmed milk, extra to allowance;
- 1 large fruit

— LUNCH —

- Sandwich of 2 slices bread with a little low-fat spread, filled with either 1 sliced medium-sized hard-boiled egg *or* 50 g (2 oz) lean cooked chicken and *unlimited* salad items
- 1 large fruit

— EVENING —

- 1 portion Potato and Ham Stir-Fry (see recipe, page 62)
- 1 diet fruit fromage frais *or* yoghurt

DAY 2

— BREAKFAST —

- 125 ml (4½ fl oz) low-fat natural yoghurt with 25 g (1 oz) dried apricots, chopped, and 1 small fruit portion mixed in

— LUNCH —

- 50 g (2 oz) corned beef *or* 75 g (3 oz) lean ham; 1 slice bread with a little low-fat spread; 75 g (3 oz) low-calorie coleslaw; *unlimited* salad items plus 1 tomato

— EVENING —

- 1 portion Meat-free Bolognese (see recipe variation, page 58), served with 50 g (2 oz) [dry weight] spaghetti, boiled, and green salad garnish from *unlimiteds*

DAY 3

—— BREAKFAST ——

• 1 slice toast, topped with either 175 g (6 oz) sliced mushrooms, microwaved in a little vegetable stock for 30 seconds *or* 3 tomatoes, halved and grilled

• 1 small fruit

—— LUNCH ——

• 75 g (3 oz) hummus; 2 rye crispbreads; selection of crudités (e.g., strips of pepper, carrot, cauliflower, onion)

1 large fruit

—— EVENING ——

• Potato omelette: beat 2 medium-sized eggs with a little water, mixed herbs and seasoning to taste; cook in non-stick frying pan in 7g (1/4 oz) low-fat spread. When nearly cooked add 200 g (7 oz) cooked chopped potato. Brown top of omelette under grill; add salad greens to garnish

or

• Homemade pizza (serves 2): top one Boboti pizza base with contents of half a jar of pizza topping; add sliced onion, peppers, mushrooms and 50 g (2 oz) chopped Mozzarella cheese; salad garnish

DAY 4

—— BREAKFAST ——

• 1 small fruit

• 25 g (1 oz) oat bran flakes or bran flakes, with 100 ml (3 1/2 fl oz) skimmed milk, extra to allowance

—— LUNCH ——

• 1 portion Potato Soup (see recipe, page 58) *or* 425 g (15 oz) can lentil soup *or* 225 g (8 oz) can baked beans in tomato sauce

• 2 slices bread or toast

—— EVENING ——

• 1 portion Prawn and Mushroom Risotto (see recipe, page 59), served with *unlimited* green salad items plus 1 tomato

DAY 5

—— BREAKFAST ——

• 125 ml (4 1/2 fl oz) low-fat natural yoghurt, with 1 large fruit and 25 g (1 oz) dried chopped apricot mixed in

—— LUNCH ——

• 100 g (3 1/2 oz) vegetable terrine *or* 50 g (2 oz) mushroom pâté; 3 Slymbred slices *or* 2 rice cakes; *unlimited* green salad items

• 1 Weight Watchers low-calorie soup of choice

• 1 large fruit

—— EVENING ——

• 1 portion Savoury Minced Beef (see recipe, page 68), topped with 175 g (6 oz) instant mashed potato and baked until top is golden; 110 g (4 oz) cabbage or courgettes; 50 g (2 oz) peas

or

• Quarterpounder extra-lean beefburger, grilled, served in 1 wholemeal bap with a little low-fat spread, *unlimited* salad garnish and 1 tsp burger relish

DAY 6

—— BREAKFAST ——

• 1 medium banana mashed with a little lemon juice and cinnamon, served on 1 slice toast with a little low-fat spread

—— LUNCH ——

• 225 g (8 oz) can wholemeal spaghetti in tomato sauce, served on 1 slice toast

• 1 large fruit

—— EVENING ——

• 1 portion Chicken Brochettes (see recipe, page 67), served with 50 g (2 oz) [dry weight] long-grain rice, boiled, and green salad garnish from *unlimiteds*

DAY 7

—— BREAKFAST ——

• 1 medium-sized egg, boiled
• 1 slice bread with a little low-fat spread

—— LUNCH ——

• Sandwich of 2 slices bread, filled with 100 g (3½ oz) low-fat cottage cheese and *unlimited* salad items plus 1 tomato
• 1 small fruit

—— EVENING ——

• 1 portion Red Pepper Pasta (see recipe, page 61), with green salad garnish from *unlimiteds*

or

• 75 g (3 oz) [dry weight] tagliatelle, served with 1 portion Tomato Sauce (see recipe, page 57) and 1 tbsp Parmesan cheese

DIET FOUR
FLEXIDIET

Many people prefer a set diet when they are slimming; however, your lifestyle – or perhaps your food preferences – may mean that you prefer to choose your own daily menus. In this case, every day choose a breakfast, a lunch and an evening meal from the following lists. The total calorie content of the meals will be approximately the same as the set diet. Extra snacks, unlimiteds and fruits remain unchanged.

—— BREAKFASTS ——
(approximately 150 calories each)

Cold

• 1 small fruit; 15g (½ oz) Puffed Wheat, with 100 ml (3½ fl oz) skimmed milk, extra to allowance
• 1½ slices bread with a little low-fat spread and 2 tsp pure fruit spread
• 125 ml (4½ fl oz) low-fat natural yoghurt, with 25 g (1 oz) chopped dried apricots
• 1 diet fruit yoghurt; 1 large banana
• 1 diet fruit fromage frais; 1 slice bread with a little low-fat spread and 1 tsp pure fruit spread
• 25 g (1 oz) bran flakes, with 50 ml (2 fl oz) skimmed milk, extra to allowance (plus extra milk from allowance, if necessary); 1 small fruit

Hot

• Porridge made from 25 g (1 oz) instant porridge oats made with half and half water and skimmed milk; 1 level tsp brown sugar
• 1 slice toast with a little low-fat spread, topped with 75 g (3 oz) baked beans
• 1 medium-sized egg, boiled or poached; 1 slice toast with a little low-fat spread
• 1 slice toast with a little low-fat spread, topped with 2 tomatoes, halved and grilled

—— LUNCHES ——
(approximately 300 calories each)

Hot

• 425 g (8 oz) can lentil soup, with 50g (2 oz) French bread *or* 2 slices bread with a little low-fat spread
• 225 g (8 oz) can baked beans on 1 slice toast with a little low-fat spread
• 1 portion Potato *or* Pea Soup (see recipe, page 58); 1½ slices bread with a little low-fat spread; 1 small fruit
• 1 Weight Watchers French Bread Pizza; 1 large fruit
• 213 g (7½ oz) can wholewheat spaghetti on 2 slices toast with a little low-fat spread
• 200 g (7 oz) baked potato, topped with 25 g (1 oz) grated reduced-fat Cheddar cheese; 1 large fruit

Cold (Salads)

• 1 portion Rice Salad with Tuna (see recipe, page 60); 1 small fruit
• Large salad of various *unlimited* items and 1 chopped tomato, mixed with 2 slices garlic sausage, chopped, and 1 medium-sized hard-boiled egg, chopped; all tossed in oil-free salad dressing; 1 slice bread with a little low-fat spread

KILL THOSE EXCUSES

Here are the top excuses overweight people use to eat more than they need to. Tick which apply to you, and vow to recognise them for what they are – excuses:

- ☐ I only bought those biscuits (substitute your own food weakness) for the children.
- ☐ I made too much food and I hate waste, so I ate it.
- ☐ I'm cooking this cake because we have guests coming.
- ☐ I ate the cake because the guests cancelled.
- ☐ How can I say 'no' when someone has been kind enough to offer me such a treat?
- ☐ I didn't have time to work out a proper meal.
- ☐ It's quicker to eat this pasty than to pick up something healthy.
- ☐ I've been good for days ...
- ☐ He/she *made* me eat/drink it.

Cold (Packed Lunches)

• Any Boots Shapers sandwich of choice; 1 large fruit or 1 diet fruit yoghurt

• Sandwich of 2 slices bread spread with a little reduced-calorie mayonnaise, filled with 100 g (3½ oz) can tuna in brine, drained and flaked, and *unlimited* salad items; 1 small fruit

• Sandwich of 2 slices bread, filled with 50 g (2 oz) lean cooked chicken – tossed in 1 tbsp low-fat natural yoghurt mixed with 1 level tsp tikka paste – and *unlimited* salad items; 1 small fruit

• 40 g (1½ oz) Brie; 3 rye crispbreads with a little low-fat spread; 1 tomato; 1 small fruit; 1 diet fromage frais

• Sandwich of 100 g (3½ oz) cottage cheese *or* 75g (3 oz) peeled prawns, and *unlimited* salad items in 2 slices bread with a little low-fat spread; 1 small fruit

• 1 wholemeal bap with a little low-fat spread, filled with 50 g (2 oz) lean ham, 1 tomato and *unlimited* salad items; 1 large fruit

—— EVENING MEALS ——

(approximately 400 calories each)

Quick and Easy

• 2 low-fat beefburgers, grilled; 200 g (7 oz) mashed potato; 75 g (3 oz) peas; thin gravy made from stock cube *or* 2 tsp relish

• 1 turkey breast steak, grilled; 200 g (7 oz) new potatoes; 75 g (3 oz) sweetcorn *or* 1 large fruit

• 175 g (6 oz) white fish steak, grilled or baked; 1 grilled potato waffle; 2 grilled tomatoes; 50 g (2 oz) peas; 1 large banana

• 1 small chicken breast fillet, skinned and coated with a mixture of 2 tbsp low-fat natural yoghurt and 2 tsp Tandoori powder, grilled or baked; *unlimited* salad items; 40 g (1½ oz) [dry weight] long-grain rice, boiled

• 110 g (4 oz) roast chicken (no skin), 375 g (13 oz) can Buitoni ratatouille, heated; 140 g (5 oz) new potatoes

• 100g (3½ oz) ham steak, grilled; 1 pineapple ring; 1 potato waffle, grilled; 75 g (3 oz) peas, sweetcorn or broad beans; 1 large banana

• 75 g (3 oz) lamb's liver, grilled with 1 small onion, sliced and stir-fried in 1 tsp oil; 175 g (6 oz) instant mashed potato; 110g (3½ oz) green beans or broccoli

Recipe Dishes

• 1 portion Chilli Chicken with Aromatic Rice (see recipe, page 66); green salad

• 1 portion Chicken and Broccoli in Yellow Bean Sauce (see recipe, page 66) with 5 tbsp (cooked weight) long-grain rice, boiled; green salad garnish from *unlimiteds*

• 1 portion Potato and Ham Stir-Fry (see recipe, page 62); 1 large fruit

• 1 portion Haddock and Spinach Layer (see recipe, page 65); 110 g (4 oz) instant mashed potato; green salad garnish from *unlimiteds*

• 1 portion Thai Chicken (see recipe, page 67); 25 g (1 oz) [dry weight] egg noodles, soaked according to manufacturer's instructions

• 1 portion cottage pie, made from 1 portion

Savoury Minced Beef (see recipe, page 68) topped with 140 g (5 oz) mashed potato; 110 g (4 oz) peas or baked beans
• 1 portion Pork and Pineapple Stir-Fry (see recipe, page 69); 25 g (1 oz) [dry weight] long-grain rice, boiled

Vegetarian meals

• 1 portion Macaroni and Chick Peas (see recipe, page 61); 1 small fruit
• 1 portion Nut Pilaff (see recipe, page 60); green salad garnish from *unlimiteds*
• 1 Marks and Spencer Vegetable and Pasta Bake; 1 slice bread with a little low-fat spread; 1 small fruit
• 225 g (8 oz) baked potato, topped with 110 g (4 oz) baked beans and 25 g (1 oz) grated reduced-fat Cheddar cheese; 1 large fruit
• 75 g (3 oz) [dry weight] tagliatelle, boiled and topped with 2 tbsp pesto or 1 portion Tomato Sauce (see recipe, page 57), plus 2 tsp Parmesan cheese; green salad garnish from *unlimiteds*
• 1 Vegetarian Feasts Tasty Lentil Bake; 1 large fruit
• 1 Vegetarian Feasts Vegetable Chilli; 40 g ($1^1/_2$ oz) [dry weight] long-grain rice, boiled

Ready-made Meals

NB: Try to limit ready-made meals to a maximum of two a week.

• 1 Marks and Spencer Filled Green Peppers; *unlimited* salad items; 1 large banana
• 1 Birds Eye Menu Master Prawn Curry and Rice; *unlimited* salad items plus 1 tomato *or* 1 small fruit
• Healthy Options Lean Beef Casserole; 1 large fruit
• 1 Birds Eye Menu Master Seafood and Chicken Paella; 1 large fruit

End of Diet 4:

Today I weigh .... st .... lbs (......... kg)

I have lost a total of .... lbs (......... kg)

since the beginning of the diet.

Re-assessment

Before you continue with your weight-loss diet, turn back to pages 22–23 and re-assess whether or not you need to lose more weight, by answering Tests 4, 5 and 6. If the answer is yes, proceed to Diet 5.

DIET FIVE

IF YOU NEED TO LOSE HALF A STONE (3.2 KG) OR LESS

Checklist:

- Have you thoroughly read all the instructions on pages 25–29?
- Don't forget the extra snacks to which you are entitled (listed on page 28); again, that's three if you're High Met, two if you're Average, and one if you're Low Met.
- Don't forget the foods that are allowed in unlimited quantities each day (listed on page 29).
- Large fruit and small fruit lists appear on pages 28–29.
- Your daily skimmed milk allowance on this diet is 125 ml ($4^1/_2$ fl oz) per day for use in tea and coffee, unless mentioned otherwise within the diet.
- The set diet beings here. For more flexibility turn to the flexi diet that begins on page 52.
- Remember to stay on this diet until you are at your target weight.
- Remember to fill in all the charts, records and spaces in the boxes provided along the way; they will help form your own personal record and will be a real help in your weight-loss campaign.

MY STARTING WEIGHT IS:

.... st .... lbs (......... kg)

MY TARGET WEIGHT IS:

.... st .... lbs (......... kg)

DAY 1

—— BREAKFAST ——

• 1 Weetabix *or* 15 g (1/2 oz) Puffed Wheat, with 100 ml (3 1/2 fl oz) skimmed milk, extra to allowance
• 1 large fruit

—— LUNCH ——

• 1 wholemeal pitta bread, filled with a salad of a few stoned and halved black olives, chopped *unlimited* salad items, 50 g (2 oz) low-fat cottage cheese, oil-free salad dressing
• 1 small fruit

—— EVENING ——

• Cheesy vegetables: lightly steam or microwave a 275 g (10 oz) selection of low-calorie vegetables (e.g., carrots, cauliflower, cabbage, green beans, courgettes), toss in 75 g (3 oz) easy cheese sauce (melt down 100 g[3 1/2 oz] low-fat soft cheese); top with 1 level tbsp pine-nuts or other chopped nuts, and serve on 40 g (1 1/2 oz) [dry weight] egg noodles, soaked according to manufacturer's instructions

DAY 2

—— BREAKFAST ——

• 140 ml (5 fl oz) orange juice
• 1 diet fruit yoghurt and 25 g (1oz) dried apricots

—— LUNCH ——

• Salad of 25 g (1 oz) [dry weight] pasta shapes, boiled, cooled and mixed with 50 g (2 oz) canned, drained, red kidney beans, sliced mushrooms and 50 g (2 oz) canned, drained or frozen sweetcorn, all tossed in oil-free salad dressing and served with *unlimited* salad items
• 1 small fruit

—— EVENING ——

• 1 portion Tangy Grilled Chicken (see recipe, page 67), served with 110 g (4 oz) boiled potatoes *or* rice and 75 g (3 oz) green beans

DAY 3

—— BREAKFAST ——

• 1 1/2 slices bread with a little low-fat spread and 2 tsp low-sugar jam or marmalade

—— LUNCH ——

• Tuna pâté: 75 g (3oz) can tuna in brine, drained and mashed with seasoning and a little low-fat natural yoghurt served on 3 rye crispbreads with *unlimited* salad items
• 1 large fruit

—— EVENING ——

• 1 portion Ratatouille with Egg (see recipe, page 63)
• 1 wholemeal roll with a little low-fat spread

or

• Vegetarian omelette: beat 2 medium-sized eggs with water and seasoning; cook in 7 g (1/4 oz) low-fat spread in non-stick pan with 25 g (1 oz) sweetcorn and 50 g (2 oz) sliced mushrooms, added before folding; 1 1/2 slices bread with a little low-fat spread; large mixed salad of *unlimited* items

DAY 4

—— BREAKFAST ——

• 25 g (1 oz) Special K or corn flakes, with 75 ml (3 fl oz) skimmed milk, extra to allowance
• 1 small fruit

—— LUNCH ——

• French bread pizza (maximum 300 calories), served with *unlimited* salad items

or

• Sandwich of 2 slices bread, filled with 25 g (1 oz) reduced-fat Cheddar cheese and *unlimited* salad items

—— EVENING ——

• 50 g (2 oz) vegetable burger, grilled, *or* fish parcel (140 g [5 oz] white fish fillet, baked in foil with seasoning and lemon juice); 175 g (6 oz) boiled *or* baked potatoes; 75 g (3 oz) mixed peas and carrots

DAY 5

— BREAKFAST —

• 125 ml ($4^1/_2$ fl oz) low-fat natural yoghurt, mixed with 1 tbsp sultanas or 25 g (1 oz) dried chopped apricots with 1 tsp runny honey drizzled over

— LUNCH —

• Sandwich of 2 slices bread, filled with 1 medium-sized hard-boiled egg, sliced, and *unlimited* salad items

— EVENING —

• 50 g (2 oz) [dry weight] pasta spirals, boiled and served with 1 portion Tomato and Mushroom Sauce (see recipe variation, page 57) [cook extra pasta for tomorrow's lunch]

• 1 medium banana

DAY 6

— BREAKFAST —

• 1 slice toast with a little low-fat spread, topped with 2 large tomatoes, halved and grilled

— LUNCH —

• 25 g (1 oz) [dry weight] pasta spirals, boiled and mixed with chopped peppers, celery, mushrooms and 75 g (3 oz) peeled prawns or tuna in brine; toss in oil-free salad dressing

— EVENING —

• 200 g (7 oz) baked potato, topped with 1 portion Chilli Con Carne (see recipe, page 69) *or* 1 portion curry sauce, mixed with contents of 110 g (4 oz) can drained beans or lentils of choice (e.g., black-eye beans, chick peas or lentils) and heated; serve *unlimited* salad items with either selection

DAY 7

— BREAKFAST —

• 25 g (1 oz) muesli, with 110 ml (4 fl oz) skimmed milk, extra to daily allowance

— LUNCH —

• 2 slices bread, thinly spread with peanut butter *or* mushroom pâté and filled with *unlimited* salad items

• 1 small fruit

— EVENING —

• 1 portion Vegetable Rice (see recipe, page 60) with 50 g (2 oz) cooked chopped chicken mixed in

or

• 200 g Birds Eye Vegetable Rice with 50 g (2 oz) chopped, cooked chicken mixed in, served with *unlimited* salad items.

If you still have more weight to lose to get down to target, repeat this week's menus or the flexi diet until you get there. If you have reached your target, *congratulations*. For information about how to maintain your new weight, turn to Chapter 10.

Make a list of all the things you plan to do when you have reached your weight-loss target. Here are some ideas:

• Turn out your wardrobe and get rid of those unflattering clothes that will probably be the wrong size.
• Treat yourself to a new hairstyle. Ask your hairdresser for advice on a style that will complement your new, slim look.
• Give yourself a complete beauty treatment. If you can't stretch to a salon makeover, do it at home. Browse through magazines to learn some new make-up tips.
• Take up a new sport, or join a local exercise class. You will no longer be ashamed to show off your figure.

DIET FIVE

FLEXIDIET

Many people prefer a set diet when they are slimming; however, your lifestyle – or perhaps your food preferences – may mean that you prefer to choose your own daily menus. In this case, every day choose a breakfast, a lunch and an evening meal from the following lists. The total calorie content of the meals will be approximately the same as the set diet. Extra snacks, unlimiteds and fruits remain unchanged.

—— BREAKFASTS ——

(approximately 150 calories each)

Cold

- 1 small fruit; 25 g (1 oz) Bran Buds or All Bran, with 110 ml (4 fl oz) skimmed milk, extra to daily allowance
- 125 ml ($4^1/_2$ fl oz) low-fat natural yoghurt mixed with 2 tsp raisins or sultanas, and 1 small chopped apple
- 1 slice bread with a little low-fat spread and 1 tsp low-sugar jam or marmalade; 1 small fruit
- 25 g (1 oz) Special K or Fruit 'n Fibre, with 110 ml (4 fl oz) skimmed milk, extra to daily allowance
- 125 ml ($4^1/_2$ fl oz) low-fat natural yoghurt, with 15 g ($^1/_2$ oz) muesli and 1 small fruit mixed in
- 15 g ($^1/_2$ oz) Puffed Wheat, with 100 ml ($3^1/_2$ fl oz) skimmed milk, extra to daily allowance; 1 large fruit
- 1 diet fruit yoghurt; 1 large banana

Hot

- 1 slice toast with a little low-fat spread, topped with 75 g (3 oz) baked beans
- 1 slice toast with a little low-fat spread, topped with 1 medium banana mashed with a little lemon juice and cinnamon
- 1 medium-sized egg, boiled or poached; 1 slice toast with a little low-fat spread
- 1 slice toast, topped with 140 g (5 oz) mushrooms, baked or microwaved with lemon juice, seasoning and 7 g ($^1/_4$ oz) low-fat spread
- 1 slice toast with a little low-fat spread, topped with 2 halved tomatoes, grilled

—— LUNCHES ——

(approximately 250 calories each)

Hot

- 1 Weight Watchers French Bread Pizza; *unlimited* green salad items
- $1^1/_2$ slices toast with a little low-fat spread, topped with 175 g (6 oz) baked beans
- 1 medium-sized poached egg on 1 slice toast with a little low-fat spread; 1 medium banana
- 200 g (7 oz) baked potato, topped with 50 g (2 oz) low-fat soft cheese, mixed with 2 chopped dates; *unlimited* green salad items
- 375 g (13 oz) can Buitoni ratatouille, heated and topped with 1 poached egg *or* 25 g (1 oz) grated reduced-fat Cheddar cheese; 1 small fruit

Cold (Salads)

- 1 wholemeal pitta bread; 50 g (2 oz) low-fat cottage cheese, mixed with 4 stoned black olives, 1 chopped tomato, 2 chopped spring onions, chopped crisp lettuce and 50 g (2 oz) finely chopped green pepper; all tossed in oil-free salad dressing
- 25 g (1 oz) [dry weight] pasta shapes, boiled and mixed with 100 g ($3^1/_2$ oz) sliced raw button mushrooms, 50 g (2 oz) red pepper, chopped, 1 small apple, chopped, 1 stick celery, chopped, and 75 g (3 oz) peeled prawns; all tossed in oil-free salad dressing

Cold (Packed Lunches)

- 2 slices bread, filled with a tuna pâté: mix 100 g ($3^1/_2$ oz) can tuna in brine, drained, with 1 tbsp low-fat natural fromage frais, and season to taste; chopped lettuce and cucumber
- Tuna pâté (as above) on 3 rye crispbreads; 1 sachet instant low-calorie soup of choice *or* 1 diet fruit yoghurt; 1 tomato

• Sandwich of 2 slices bread, spread thinly with reduced-calorie mayonnaise and filled with 1 medium-sized egg, hard-boiled and sliced, and *unlimited* salad items.
• 2 slices bread spread with yeast extract and filled with *unlimited* salad items; 1 medium banana *or* 1 diet fruit yoghurt and 1 small fruit
• Sandwich of 2 slices bread with a little low-fat spread, filled with 50 g (2 oz) lean ham and *unlimited* salad items
• 1 small cooked chicken portion, with skin removed; 2 rye crispbreads with a little low-fat spread; 1 tomato; 1 small fruit

—— EVENING MEALS ——

(approximately 350 calories each)

Quick and Easy

• 110 g (4 oz) peeled prawns, heated in 175 g (6 oz) ready-made Indian curry sauce with vegetables; 5 tbsp (cooked weight) long-grain rice, boiled; *unlimited* green salad items
• 100 g (3½ oz) chicken fillet, skin removed, brushed with Hoi Sin sauce, and grilled or baked, in 1 wholemeal bap with *unlimited* side salad
• 1 portion fish in parsley sauce (frozen), 175 g (6 oz) baked, boiled or instant mashed potatoes; 75g (3 oz) peas
• 1 portion cod in wholemeal breadcrumbs (frozen), baked or grilled; 1 potato waffle, baked or grilled; 100 g (3½ oz) green beans or broccoli
• 2 low-fat pork chipolatas, grilled; 150 g (5½ oz) instant mashed potato; 150 g (5½ oz) baked beans
• 1 McCain or McVitie Pizza Slice; large side salad of *unlimited* items; 1 large banana
• 75 g (3 oz) lean roast beef, cut into strips and stir-fried with 100g (3½ oz) chopped red pepper and 2 tbsp ready-made black bean sauce; 40 g (1½ oz) [dry weight] long-grain rice, boiled
• 1 Findus Sliced Roast Beef with Gravy; 150 g (5½ oz) boiled or baked potatoes; 150 g (5½ oz) cabbage
• 110 g (4 oz) chicken portion, baked or grilled *or* 110 g (4 oz) roast chicken (no skin); 150 g (5½ oz) boiled or baked potatoes; 110 g (4 oz) mixed peas and carrots; a little thin gravy made from stock cube

Recipe Dishes

• 1 portion Chicken Brochettes (see recipe, page 67); 40 g (1½ oz) [dry weight] long-grain rice, boiled; green salad garnish from *unlimiteds*
• 1 portion Chilli Con Carne (see recipe, page 69) with 175 g (6 oz) baked potato *or* 40 g (1½ oz) [dry weight] long-grain rice, boiled
• 1 portion Nutty Chicken with Beansprouts (see recipe, page 68); 25 g (1 oz) [dry weight] egg noodles, soaked according to manufacturer's instructions; green salad garnish from *unlimiteds*
• 2 Tuna Fish Cakes (see recipe, page 64); 75 g (3 oz) peas; 110 g (4 oz) broccoli
• 1 portion Tangy Grilled Chicken (see recipe, page 67); 150 g (5½ oz) new potatoes; large salad of *unlimiteds* plus 1 tomato
• 1 portion Tandoori Fish Kebabs (see recipe, page 64); 6 tbsp (cooked weight) long-grain rice, boiled; *unlimited* green salad garnish
• 1 portion Sweet and Sour Stir-Fry (see recipe, page 65); 5 tbsp (cooked weight) long-grain rice, boiled

Vegetarian Meals

• 1 portion Ratatouille with Egg (see recipe, page 63); 1 small wholemeal roll
• 300 g (10½ oz) vegetable lasagne (ready-made: maximum 210 calories); *unlimited* salad items; 1 large banana
• 1 portion Vegetable Rice (see recipe, page 60); *unlimited* salad items; 1 medium banana
• 50 g (2 oz) [dry weight] pasta of choice, boiled and topped with 1 portion Tomato and Mushroom Sauce (see recipe variation, page 57); 2 tsp Parmesan cheese; *unlimited* salad items; 1 small fruit
• 200 g (7 oz) baked potato with 200 g (7 oz) can chilli beans; *unlimited* salad items
• 4 crispy vegetable fingers (ready-made: maximum 50 calories each), grilled or baked; 150 g (5½ oz) new potatoes; 75 g (3oz) green beans; 1 small fruit
• Vegetarian shepherd's pie (ready-made: maximum 300 calories); 1 large fruit
• Vegetarian Moussaka (ready-made: maximum 300 calories); large salad of *unlimited* items *or* 1 small fruit

Ready-made Meals

NB: Try to limit ready-made meals to a maximum of two a week.

- Spaghetti Bolognese (maximum 300 calories); 1 large fruit
- Findus Lean Cuisine Glazed Chicken with Vegetable Rice; large salad of *unlimited* items, plus 1 tomato; 1 large fruit
- Findus Lean Cuisine Chilli Con Carne; large salad of *unlimited* items, plus 1 tomato; 1 large fruit

Date started on Diet 5: ....

Weight on starting:......... st ....lbs (......... kg)

Date reached target weight: ....

Target weight is: .... st .... lbs (......... kg)

Statistics at target weight:

Bust/chest: .... ins (.........cm) Waist: .... ins (......... cm) Hips: .... ins (......... cm)

Feelings

Now I have reached my target weight, I feel: ....

....

To celebrate I am going to: ....

....

6 The Speed Plus Plan

The Speed Plus Plan is a short-term diet, with only 800 calories allowed each day. The main use for this diet is to get you back on course when your best-laid dieting plans have gone wrong. If you have had a binge, eaten more than you should have, or had two consecutive days of socialising, eating out, snacking or eating many foods that aren't on your diet plan, you can spend two days on the Speed Plus Plan to get yourself back on course. It's the physical and psychological boost you need to resume your diet successfully.

You should *never* follow the Speed Plus Plan for more than five days at a time – but this should be more than adequate. Usually, the diet should only be needed one or two days at a time.

The Speed Plus Plan can also be used after you have reached your target weight, and have transferred to the Maintenance Plan (see Chapter 10). Before or after a 'food-indulgent day', you can follow the diet to make sure your weight remains stable.

Instructions

There are four food groups on the Speed Plus Plan. All you do is choose one 'mini meal' from each group every day and evenly space the meals out throughout the day. If you are on the diet for more than one day, vary your choices as much as possible.

Large and small fruit choices are the same as in the sliding-scale diets on pages 28–29. *Unlimited* foods on the diet are also the same, listed on page 29.

Only water, mineral water, fruit or herbal teas, or weak black tea or coffee may be drunk.

Food Groups

Group 1

- 100 g (3½ oz) low-fat cottage or soft cheese; 3 rye crispbreads; 1 large tomato
- Sandwich of 2 slices low-calorie bread filled with 75 g (3 oz) low-fat soft cheese and *unlimited* salad items
- 1 small wholemeal roll, with a little low-fat spread, filled with 25 g (1 oz) grated reduced-fat Cheddar, tomato and celery
- 1 diet fruit yoghurt; 25 g (1 oz) dried apricots *or* peaches
- 25 g (1 oz) muesli with 125 ml (4½ fl oz) low-fat natural yoghurt
- Milkshake made from 225 ml (8 fl oz) skimmed milk, blended with 25 ml (1 fl oz) orange juice and 1 small banana, plus a pinch of cinnamon
- 1 tub fruit fromage frais; 1 banana
- 125 ml (4½ fl oz) low-fat natural yoghurt, with 2 large fruit chopped in

Group 2

- 1 average wholemeal bread roll with a little low-fat spread; 2 tsp low-sugar jam *or* marmalade; 1 large fruit
- 2 slices bread with a little low-fat spread and yeast extract; 1 large fruit
- 1 wholemeal pitta; 2 tbsp low-fat natural yoghurt mixed with chopped cucumber and mint; 1 small fruit
- 1 mini wholemeal pitta bread; 40 g (1½ oz) hummus; 1 large fruit
- 50 g (2 oz) French bread; 15 g (½ oz) vegetable spread; 1 tomato

- 213 g ($7^1/_2$ oz) can wholewheat spaghetti in tomato sauce on 1 slice toast with a little low-fat spread
- 25 g (1 oz) mushroom spread on 1 slice toast with a little low-fat spread; 1 large fruit
- 1 can Weight Watchers Low-Calorie Vegetable Soup; 1 small wholemeal roll with a little low-fat spread; 1 small fruit
- 1 large banana, mashed, on $1^1/_2$ slices toast with a little low-fat spread
- 40 g ($1^1/_2$ oz) muesli, with 140 ml (5 fl oz) skimmed milk
- 25 g (1 oz) All Bran or Bran Buds, with 75 ml (3 fl oz) skimmed milk; 1 medium banana
- 25 g (1 oz) Special K or Fruit 'n Fibre, with 110 ml (4 fl oz) skimmed milk and 1 large fruit

Group 3

- 50 g (2 oz) peeled prawns and 50 g (2 oz) sliced raw mushrooms, mixed with 75 g (3 oz) [cooked weight] pasta, boiled, and oil-free salad dressing
- 175 g (6 oz) baked potato with 7 g ($^1/_4$ oz) butter *or* 15 g ($^1/_2$ oz) low-fat spread
- 50 g (2 oz) grilled vegetable burger with 1 tsp relish; 100 g ($3^1/_2$ oz) instant mashed potato
- 50 g (2oz) cooked lean chicken; 100 g ($3^1/_2$ oz) instant mashed potato; medium serving broccoli *or* green beans
- 2 wholemeal crumb-coated cod or haddock fish fingers, grilled; 100 g ($3^1/_2$ oz) instant mashed potato; 75 g (3 oz) carrot
- 1 slice toast with a little low-fat spread; 150 g ($5^1/_2$ oz) baked beans in tomato sauce
- 275 g (10 oz) can low-calorie vegetable soup; 1 slice bread with a little low-fat spread
- 1 medium-sized egg, boiled or poached; 1 slice bread with a little low-fat spread; 1 small fruit

Group 4

- 1 large banana; 1 large fruit; 1 rye crispbread with a little low fat spread
- Large mixed salad with oil-free salad dressing *or* lemon juice; 1 medium-sized egg, hard-boiled, and 1 rye crispbread
- Selection of crudités; 50 g (2 oz) low-fat natural yoghurt, with chopped cucumber and mint; 1 large banana
- Large portion fresh beansprouts, raw or lightly steamed, and topped with 1 tbsp soya sauce; 1 large banana
- Coleslaw: toss shredded white cabbage, carrot, finely chopped onion and 1 tbsp sultanas in a mixture of 1 tbsp low-fat natural yoghurt and 2 tsp reduced-calorie mayonnaise
- Sweet and sour salad: roughly chop lettuce leaves (lollo rosso and frisee if you can find them) with chicory leaves and watercress, and toss with 1 orange, segmented. Mix 1 tsp runny honey with 2 tsp wine or balsamic vinegar, and sprinkle over salad
- Fruit and nut salad: mix 2 large or 3 small fruit (chopped as necessary) and sprinkle with 20 g ($^3/_4$ oz) flaked, toasted almonds

7 Speed Slimming Recipes

All of the recipes in this chapter appear in the sliding-scale diets. You can also use them on your maintenance diet, when you have reached your target weight. The recipes can be enjoyed by dieters and non-dieters alike so there's no need to cook separate meals.

In most cases, each recipe serves two people, but the quantities can be halved very easily to serve one, or doubled to serve four. If you eat alone, bear in mind that many of the recipes can be frozen, so it is worth making a double quantity and using the frozen portion the next time that particular meal appears in your diet or maintenance plan.

The recipes require only moderate cooking skills, but they're interesting and tasty. Most are quick to prepare, and their costs have been kept quite low by using inexpensive ingredients – with the very occasional luxury!

Most ingredients will be familiar to you; some may not. I urge you to give dishes you've never tried before a chance; a healthy diet is comprised of a variety of *different* foods and acquiring new tastes will not only expand your culinary repertoire, but it will make you feel better, too. When there's lots to choose from, the possibility of boredom diminishes, so give them a try!

So, whenever possible, try to vary your diet from day to day. Unless it is a summer heatwave, when you might not feel like eating hot food, try to ensure that you also vary the *type* of meals you choose. In other words, don't select a fruit for breakfast, a salad for lunch and then another salad for your evening meal, day after day, or you will become very bored (even though you may not consciously be aware of this). If you stick to a 'salads only' diet, before long you will probably find yourself yearning for a forbiddden food, when in fact by varying your diet to include fish, meat or a hot pasta dish, for instance, you will prevent your body craving for something that you shouldn't eat.

SOUPS & SAUCES

TOMATO SAUCE

(MAKES 4 SERVINGS OF APPROXIMATELY 70 CALORIES EACH)

1 tbsp corn or olive oil
1 Spanish onion, very finely chopped
Dash white wine *or* white wine vinegar
275 g (10 oz) Passata (sieved tomatoes)
1 tsp garlic purée
1 tbsp tomato purée
Pinch brown sugar
Dash soya sauce
1 tsp dried *or* 2 tsp fresh chopped basil
Little salt and black pepper

Heat the oil in a frying pan and sauté the onion over medium heat until soft. Add the wine or vinegar, let it bubble, then add all the remaining ingredients, stirring well. Allow to simmer for ten minutes.

Variation

- Add 100 g (3½ oz) sliced mushrooms to the recipe, before simmering.
- Add a dash of chilli seasoning for a hot tomato sauce.
- Add a couple of skinned, chopped tomatoes for more texture.

CURRY SAUCE

(MAKES 4 SERVINGS OF APPROXIMATELY 65 CALORIES EACH)

1 tbsp corn or olive oil
1 strong-flavoured onion, finely chopped
2 tsp mild or medium curry powder, to taste
400 g (14 oz) can chopped tomatoes
1 vegetable or chicken stock cube
1 heaped tsp cornflour
Little salt

Heat the oil in a frying pan and sauté the onion until just turning golden. Add the curry powder, stir well and cook for 1 minute. Add the tomatoes and simmer for a few minutes.

Mix stock cube in 100 ml (3½ fl oz) boiling water; blend cornflour in very little water and stir into stock. Add the stock/cornflour blend to the pan and stir gently.

Allow the sauce to simmer, stirring continuously, until thick. Add a little salt.

• If you're on the maintenance diet, use two portions of this sauce (half the recipe) and add some cooked chopped chicken or vegetables; and serve with rice or a baked potato for a filling main meal for one.

SPEEDY BOLOGNESE SAUCE

(MAKES 4 SERVINGS OF 210 CALORIES EACH)

325 g (12 oz) extra-lean minced beef
1 large green pepper, de-seeded and finely chopped *or* 175 g (6 oz) mushrooms, chopped
1 beef stock cube
1 quantity Tomato Sauce (see recipe, page 57)

Place the meat in a non-stick frying pan over a medium heat, and cook until brown. Add the peppers (or mushrooms) and stir until softened.

Mix beef stock cube in a little boiling water and stir into beef.

Stir in Tomato Sauce, and simmer for 10 – 20 minutes.

Variation

• For a meat-free Bolognese, omit the minced beef substituting either 225 g (8 oz) soya mince or 175 g (6 oz) brown lentils; replace stock cube with the vegetable equivalent. Simmer all ingredients together in a pan until tender (lentils can take up to 1 hour).

POTATO SOUP

(SERVES 2 AT 170 CALORIES PER PORTION)

2 tsp corn or olive oil
1 small onion, finely chopped
175 g (6 oz) potato, peeled and cubed
1 chicken or vegetable stock cube
150 ml (5½ fl oz) skimmed milk
Little salt and black pepper
10 ready-made croutons, garlic or plain
1 tbsp chopped parsley

Heat the oil in a non-stick pan and sauté the onion until transparent. Add potato and stir for about 1 minute.

Dissolve stock cube in 150 ml (5 fl oz) boiling water and add to milk. Stir stock/milk mixture into potatoes and onions and simmer for 30 minutes.

Liquidise the soup in a blender or food processor; season to taste.

Before serving, sprinkle with parsley and croutons.

Variation

• For a change, use 85 g (3 oz) potato and 85 g (3 oz) tender frozen peas or petit pois; add the peas with the stock. Garnish with chopped mint instead of parsley.

DON'T BE A DIET BORE!

If you are cooking for members of your family, they will find it easier to tolerate your slimming campaign if you do not announce each dish as being a 'diet' recipe that is good for them every time you serve it. People are often surprised to discover that low-calorie dishes can taste quite delicious – as well as being healthy – but they don't need to be reminded about it all the time!

RICE AND PASTA

TOMATO AND HAM TAGLIATELLE

(SERVES 2 AT 450 CALORIES PER PORTION)

2 tsp olive oil
1 small onion, finely chopped
1 clove garlic, chopped (optional)
175 g (6 oz) small button mushrooms, whole
1/2 quantity Tomato Sauce (see recipe, page 57) *or* 275 g (10 oz) ready-made Italian tomato sauce
50 g (2 oz) smoked ham, cut into strips
175 g (6 oz) tagliatelle, half white, half green

Heat the oil in a non-stick pan and sauté the onion until just turning golden; add the garlic (if using) and stir for 1 minute.

Add the mushrooms, tomato sauce and ham, stir and simmer for 10 minutes.

Boil the pasta in plenty of salted water according to manufacturer's instructions, drain and toss with the sauce.

Garnish with any fresh herbs or watercress as available.

PRAWN AND MUSHROOM RISOTTO

(SERVES 2 AT 375 CALORIES PER PORTION)

2 tsp corn or olive oil
15 g (1/2 oz) butter
1 small onion, finely chopped
1 clove garlic, finely chopped
Pinch turmeric (or mild curry powder)
110 g (4 oz) risotto or long-grain rice
500 ml (18 fl oz) fish stock, from cube
110 g (4 oz) mushrooms, sliced
25 g (1 oz) frozen sweetcorn
110 g (4 oz) peeled, cooked prawns
Little salt and black pepper
Chopped parsley

Heat the oil and butter in a non-stick frying pan and stir the onion until transparent. Add garlic and turmeric, stir for another minute more.

Add the rice and stir-fry for about 3 minutes.

Add sweetcorn, stock and a little seasoning, bring to a simmer; cover pan and simmer until liquid is nearly absorbed – about 20 minutes. (If rice looks too dry during cooking, add a little water.)

Five minutes before the end of cooking time, add the mushrooms and stir. Just before serving, stir in the prawns.

When all liquid is absorbed, taste for seasoning and serve garnished with chopped parsley.

Variation

- Use 110 g (4 oz) tuna in brine instead of prawns.
- Vegetarians, substitute diced tofu for prawns, and vegetable stock for fish stock.

CHOW MEIN

(SERVES 2 AT 425 CALORIES PER PORTION)

125 g (41/2 oz) dried egg noodles
2 tsp corn oil
4 spring onions, halved
1 small red pepper, de-seeded and sliced
1 small carrot, cut into strips
2 tsp dry sherry (optional)
1 tbsp soya sauce
40 g (11/2 oz) flaked toasted almonds

Soak the noodles according to manufacturer's instructions and drain.

Heat the oil and stir-fry the onion, pepper and carrot for 3 minutes.

Add sherry, soya sauce and bring to a bubble for 30 seconds.

Add noodles, and nuts; stir and serve.

Variation

- For a moister noodle dish, add 50 ml (2 fl oz) chicken stock with the soya sauce.
- Stock from a cube will only add 7 calories per portion.

RICE SALAD WITH TUNA

(SERVES 2 AT 255 CALORIES PER PORTION)

- 75 g (3 oz) long-grain rice
- 1 small onion, finely chopped
- 1 small red pepper, de-seeded and chopped
- 2 tsp olive oil
- 50 g (2 oz) mushrooms, sliced
- 25 g (1 oz) tender frozen peas
- 185 g (6½ oz) tuna in brine, drained and flaked
- Chopped parsley

Boil the rice in salted water until tender, adding peas for last few minutes. Drain if necessary, and set aside.

Heat the oil and stir-fry the onion, pepper and mushrooms in a small non-stick pan until just soft.

Stir together the rice, peas, vegetables and tuna, and garnish with parsley.

VEGETABLE RICE

(SERVES 2 AT 240 CALORIES PER PORTION)

- 2 tsp corn oil
- 4 spring onions, halved
- 1 medium carrot, cut into small cubes
- 1 medium yellow pepper, de-seeded and chopped
- 50 g (2 oz) frozen peas
- 200 g (7 oz) cooked long-grain rice
- 1 medium egg, beaten
- 1 tbsp soya sauce
- Salt and pepper to taste

Heat the oil in a non-stick pan and stir-fry the onions, carrot and pepper for 3 minutes.

Add remainder of ingredients and stir-fry until egg is cooked.

Variation

• Almost any low calorie vegetable can be added to this dish. You can also add spices of your choice – a little ginger or turmeric is nice.
• For a moister dish, add a little vegetable stock thickened, if necessary, with cornflour.

NUT PILAFF

(SERVES 2 AT 400 CALORIES PER PORTION)

- 75 g (3 oz) long-grain or brown rice
- 2 tsp corn oil
- 7 g (¼ oz) butter
- 1 small onion, finely chopped
- 1 small green pepper, de-seeded and chopped
- 50 g (2 oz) courgettes, finely chopped
- 50 g (2 oz) button mushrooms, sliced
- 50 g (2 oz) shelled cashew nuts
- 2 tsp mushroom ketchup
- 1 level tsp ground cumin
- 50 ml (2 fl oz) vegetable or chicken stock from cube
- Little salt and black pepper

Boil the rice in salted water until tender, drain if necessary and set aside.

Heat butter and oil in non-stick frying pan; fry onion until just turning golden. Add pepper and courgettes and stir-fry for further 2 to 3 minutes. Add mushrooms, stir-fry for 1 minute.

Add rest of ingredients, plus the rice, and simmer for a few minutes to heat through.

CHEESY CHICKEN AND PASTA

(SERVES 2 AT 450 CALORIES PER PORTION)

- 110 g (4 oz) pasta spirals (or shape of choice)
- 1 medium green pepper, de-seeded and chopped
- 2 tsp corn oil
- 175 g (6 oz) chicken-breast meat, skinned and cut into slices
- 1 small onion, sliced into thin rings
- 1 leek, sliced into rounds
- 1 medium carrot, cut into strips
- 1 clove garlic, chopped
- 1 level tsp Mediterranean herbs
- Little salt and black pepper
- 50 g (2 oz) Italian Mozzarella cheese,chopped

Boil the pasta in salted water according to manufacturer's instructions. Drain and set aside.

Heat the oil in a non-stick pan and stir-fry the chicken slices over a medium heat until cooked and golden. Remove from the pan.

Stir-fry the onion, pepper, leeks and carrot, adding a little chicken stock if the pan gets too dry, until all vegetables are cooked, but still crisp.

Return pasta and chicken to pan, adding the garlic, herbs and seasoning, and stir gently to heat through.

Add the Mozzarella cheese, stir to melt slightly, and serve.

RED PEPPER PASTA

(SERVES 2 AT 400 CALORIES PER PORTION)

1 tbsp olive oil

Half a Spanish onion, thinly sliced

1 clove garlic, chopped

2 rashers lean-cut back bacon, cut into strips

2 medium red peppers, de-seeded and thickly sliced

10 stoned black olives, halved

200 g (7 oz) can chopped tomatoes with herbs

Dash red wine

Little salt and black pepper

110 g (4 oz) ribbon pasta

1 tbsp grated Parmesan cheese

Heat the oil in a non-stick frying pan and sauté the onion until transparent. Add the garlic and bacon and cook until bacon is crisp, and the onion golden.

Turn down heat and add the peppers. Stir-fry until soft.

Add olives, wine and seasoning and bring to a bubble.

Add tomatoes and simmer for 15 minutes. Meanwhile, boil the pasta in salted water according to manufacturer's instructions. Drain, toss with sauce, serve with cheese sprinkled over.

• Rinse black olives well in cold running water to reduce saltiness. Choose the largest black olives you can find; they usually have the best taste.

Variation

• Vegetarians can omit the bacon and add 1 extra tbsp Parmesan cheese per serving.
• If you prefer, instead of the bacon you can substitute any left-over cooked meats (perhaps chicken or lamb) from a previous meal, or use chopped ham.

MACARONI AND CHICK PEAS

(SERVES 2 AT 375 CALORIES PER PORTION)

1 tbsp olive oil

1 small onion, finely chopped

1 clove garlic, chopped

1 medium carrot, cut into small chunks

1 level tsp ground coriander

200 g (7 oz) can chopped tomatoes

2 tsp tomato purée

110 g (4 oz) dried macaroni
(or other small pasta shapes)

200 g (7 oz) can chick peas, drained

Little salt and black pepper

2 tbsp Parmesan cheese

Heat the oil in a small flame-proof casserole or lidded non-stick pan and sauté the onion and garlic until soft. Add carrot and coriander and stir for 1 minute.

Add tomatoes, tomato purée, pasta, chick peas and 50 ml (2 fl oz) water, and simmer for 20 minutes, adding a little more water if necessary.

When pasta is tender and you have a rich sauce, taste for seasoning, and serve with Parmesan cheese.

Pasta is a versatile, economical food. High in complex carbohydrates, fat-free and filling, it forms an ideal part of any slimming diet. However, make sure you don't combine it with fattening creamy sauces. Quick and easy to cook, it is a boon for busy slimmers. It's always worthwhile cooking some extra pasta to have cold with a salad the next day. There are endless varieties of pasta to choose from, including vegetable ones such as spinach and tomato. Use coloured pasta or mix different shapes to add extra interest to meals. Wholewheat pasta contains valuable fibre and nutrients, so use this in preference to white pasta. Fresh pasta should be stored in a fridge and used within 24 hours of purchase. Unopened packets of dried pasta will keep for months if stored in a cool, dry place, but once opened, the packet should be used as quickly as possible.

VEGETABLE, EGG & PULSE DISHES

CHEESY VEGETABLE BAKE

(SERVES 2 AT 450 CALORIES PER PORTION)

1 tbsp olive oil
1 medium onion, chopped
1 clove garlic, chopped
250 g (9 oz) sliced par-boiled potatoes
1 medium courgette, sliced
1 red pepper, de-seeded and sliced
1/2 quantity Tomato Sauce (see recipe, page 57) *or* 200 g (7 oz) ready-made Italian tomato sauce
150 ml (5½ fl oz) vegetable stock from cube
1 level tsp mixed Mediterranean herbs
Little salt and black pepper
100 g (3½ oz) thick low-fat natural yoghurt
50 g (2 oz) Mozzarella cheese, chopped
25 g (1 oz) half-fat Cheddar cheese
25 g (1 oz) wholemeal breadcrumbs

Heat oil in a non-stick frying pan and sauté onion until soft. Add garlic and vegetables, and fry gently for 2 minutes, so the potatoes don't crumble.

Add the tomato sauce, stock and seasoning, and simmer uncovered until vegetables are tender.

Transfer mixture to ovenproof serving dish, top with yoghurt, cheese and then breadcrumbs, and brown under grill before serving.

POTATO AND HAM STIR-FRY

(SERVES 2 AT 340 CALORIES PER PORTION)

1 tbsp corn oil
400 g (14 oz) potatoes, par-boiled and sliced
1 small onion, finely chopped
1 medium courgette, chopped *or* 150 g (5½ oz) cauliflower florets
150 g (5½ oz) white cabbage, finely chopped
1 small red pepper, de-seeded and chopped
100 g (3½ oz) smoked ham, sliced
Little salt and black pepper
1 tbsp chopped parsley

Heat the oil in a non-stick frying pan and add the potatoes and onion, stir-frying for a few minutes.

Add the pepper, courgette and cabbage, and stir-fry for a further 3 minutes.

Add the ham and seasoning and fry for another minute. Finally, stir in the parsley and serve.

Variation

- Vegetarians can add 100 g (3½ oz) drained, canned red kidney beans instead of the ham.
- As a change from ham, try 50 g (2 oz) corned beef.
- For a moister dish, add 1 tsp French mustard, mixed with a little vegetable stock.

> Vegetarians should note that many of the recipes can be adapted by following the variations given throughout the chapter, or by substituting meat with tofu, for instance.

SAVOURY LENTIL CRUMBLE

(SERVES 2 AT 450 CALORIES PER PORTION)

1 tbsp corn oil
1 medium onion, finely chopped
250 g (9 oz) potatoes, peeled and diced
125 g (4½ oz) carrots, peeled and diced
1 large stick celery, chopped
50 g (2 oz) red lentils
2 tsp plain flour
1 bouquet garni
275 ml (10 fl oz) vegetable stock from cube
Little salt and black pepper
50 g (2 oz) breadcrumbs
50 g (2 oz) half-fat Cheddar cheese, grated

Heat oil in a non-stick frying pan and sauté onion until just turning golden. Add potatoes, carrot, celery and lentils, and stir.

Sprinkle flour over vegetables and stir again. Add bouquet garni, stock and seasonings, and stir, bringing to a simmer.

Simmer covered for 30 minutes, or until lentils are tender, then remove bouquet garni.

Place in an ovenproof serving dish, top with the breadcrumbs and cheese, and brown under grill.

VEGETABLE CURRY

(SERVES 2 AT 350 CALORIES PER PORTION)

1 tbsp corn oil
2 tsp mild curry powder (or to taste)
1 medium onion, chopped
2 medium carrots, peeled and sliced
275 g (10 oz) cauliflower florets
175 g (6 oz) peeled and diced potato
200 g (7 oz) can chopped tomatoes
50 g (2 oz) lentils, red or brown
50 ml (2 fl oz) vegetable stock from cube
50 ml (2 fl oz) skimmed milk
75 g (3 oz) frozen peas
1 tsp lemon juice
1 level tsp garam marsala

Heat the oil in a non-stick frying pan, add curry powder and stir to dissolve. Add onion and cook for a few minutes.

Stir in vegetables, lentils, stock and milk, and simmer for 20 minutes or until vegetables are tender. (Make sure to simmer the dish; if it fast boils the cauliflower will break up.)

Stir in the peas, lemon juice and garam marsala, and simmer for a further 3 minutes. Serve.

RATATOUILLE WITH EGG

(SERVES 2 AT 210 CALORIES PER PORTION)

1 small aubergine
2 medium courgettes, sliced
1 green or red pepper, de-seeded and sliced
1 large onion, sliced
1 clove garlic, chopped
200 g (7 oz) can tomatoes
1 tsp ground coriander *or* basil
Little salt and pepper
2 medium eggs

Cube the aubergine, place the pieces with the courgettes in a colander and sprinkle with coarse salt, to remove any bitterness. Allow to drain for 30 minutes; rinse and pat dry.

Heat oil in an ovenproof lidded casserole and sauté onion until just turning golden.

Add garlic, vegetables and seasoning, cover and simmer for 1 hour, or until all the vegetables are tender. If necessary you can add a little tomato juice or water to the pan, if it looks too dry.

When the ratatouille is cooked, make two wells in it; break an egg into each and simmer until the eggs are set – about 10 minutes.

FISH DISHES

FISH MOUSSAKA

(SERVES 2 AT 415 CALORIES PER PORTION)

275 g (10 oz) white fish fillets
275 ml (10 fl oz) skimmed milk
1 tbsp chopped parsley
Little salt and black pepper
2 tomatoes, sliced
275 g (10 oz) potatoes, boiled and sliced
15 g (½ oz) low-fat spread
15 g (½ oz) plain flour
75 g (3 oz) half-fat Cheddar cheese, grated
Pinch of paprika

Place the fish and milk in a frying pan and poach for a few minutes. Drain and reserve milk; flake fish into an ovenproof dish.

Sprinkle on some parsley and add a layer of tomatoes.

Sprinkle with salt, then add a layer of potatoes.

In a small non-stick pan, make a cheese sauce: melt the low-fat spread, add the flour and stir for 1 minute. Slowly add the reserved milk, constantly stirring until it thickens.

Add the cheese and stir until melted. Taste for seasoning.

Pour sauce over potatoes and sprinkle with paprika. Cook in a moderate oven until piping hot through (about 20 minutes) and serve with a sprinkle of parsley.

TANDOORI FISH KEBABS

(SERVES 2 AT 220 CALORIES PER PORTION)

- 1 tbsp tandoori powder
- 200 ml (7 fl oz) low-fat natural yoghurt
- 1 tbsp lemon juice
- 350 g (12½ oz) cod fillet, cubed
- 1 small onion, quartered and split
- lemon wedges (to garnish)

Mix together the tandoori powder, lemon juice and yoghurt, add the fish and leave to marinate for half an hour.

Thread the fish on two skewers, alternating with the larger outer pieces of onion.

Grill under medium heat for 10 minutes, turning once.

Serve garnished with lemon wedges.

TUNA AND BROCCOLI BAKE

(SERVES 2 AT 365 CALORIES PER PORTION)

- 300 g (11 oz) broccoli florets, lightly boiled
- 200 g (7 oz) tuna in brine, drained and flaked
- 15 g (½ oz) low-fat spread
- 15 g (½ oz) plain flour
- 275 ml (10 fl oz) skimmed milk
- Little salt and black pepper
- Pinch of mustard powder
- 75 g (3 oz) half-fat Cheddar cheese, grated
- 2 tomatoes, quartered

Arrange the broccoli florets around the edge of an ovenproof gratin dish. Arrange the tuna in the centre.

In a small non-stick pan, melt the low-fat spread and stir in the flour; cook for 1 minute, stirring all the time. Add the milk, salt, pepper and mustard powder, and stir until the sauce simmers and thickens.

Pour the sauce over the tuna and base of the broccoli, top with the grated cheese.

Arrange the tomato quarters around the edge, in between the broccoli, and bake at 400°F (200 °C, Gas mark 6) until cheese topping is light golden (about 20 minutes).

TUNA FISH CAKES

(MAKES 4 FISH CAKES AT 115 CALORIES EACH)

- 200 g (7 oz) can tuna in brine, drained
- 1 medium onion, finely chopped
- 175 g (6 oz) boiled or instant mashed potato
- 1 tsp anchovy essence (optional)
- 1 tsp capers (optional)
- 2 tsp chopped parsley
- 1 tsp Worcestershire sauce
- Little salt and black pepper
- 2 tsp flour mixed with a little salt and pepper
- 2 tsp corn oil

In a large bowl, mash and mix all the ingredients, except the flour and oil. Form into 4 cakes.

Spread the flour out on a small plate and carefully coat each cake in the flour. Brush each cake with oil. Grill or dry-fry the cakes in a non-stick pan for 5 minutes each side, over a medium heat.

Variation

• You can use any fish fillet to make these cakes; if you use salmon add approximately 25 calories per fish cake.

COD CREOLE

(SERVES 2 AT 450 CALORIES PER PORTION)

- 1 tbsp corn oil
- 1 medium onion, finely chopped
- 1 green pepper, de-seeded and chopped
- 50 g (2 oz) pineapple, chopped
- 200 g (7 oz) can chopped tomatoes
- 1 tbsp tomato purée
- 1 tsp Tabasco sauce
- 1 tsp Worcestershire sauce
- Little salt and black pepper
- 325 g (12 oz) cod fillet, cut into bite-sized pieces
- 110 g (4 oz) [dry weight] egg noodles
- Tomato juice as necessary

Heat the oil in a non-stick frying pan, and sauté the onion until soft. Add the green pepper and sauté for 3 minutes more.

Add the pineapple, tomatoes, tomato purée and seasonings, and simmer uncovered for 10 minutes.

Add the cod and simmer for a further 7 to 8 minutes, adding a little tomato juice if necessary to prevent the mixture from becoming too dry.

Meanwhile, soak the noodles according to manufacturer's instructions and blend with the cod creole to serve.

HADDOCK AND SPINACH LAYER

(SERVES 2 AT 315 CALORIES PER PORTION)

225 g (8 oz) frozen chopped spinach, defrosted
225 g (8 oz) smoked haddock fillet, cubed
15 g (½ oz) low-fat spread
15 g (½ oz) plain flour
275 ml (10 fl oz) skimmed milk
50 g (2 oz) half-fat Cheddar cheese, grated
Salt and pepper to taste
25 g (1 oz) wholemeal breadcrumbs

Spread the spinach in the base of an ovenproof dish and arrange the smoked haddock on top.

In a small non-stick pan, heat the low-fat spread and stir in the flour; cook for 1 minute then add the milk, stirring, until it simmers and thickens.

Add half the cheese and stir again. Season to taste, then pour the sauce over the fish and top with the breadcrumbs and remaining cheese. Bake at 350°F (180°C, Gas mark 4), for 30 minutes, or until top is golden.

SWEET AND SOUR STIR-FRY

(SERVES 2 AT 240 CALORIES PER PORTION)

1 tbsp runny honey
1 tbsp soya sauce
1 level tbsp tomato purée
2 tbsp white wine vinegar
2 level tsp cornflour
1 tbsp corn oil
25 ml (1 fl oz) water
4 spring onions, chopped
1 red pepper, de-seeded and chopped
175 g (6 oz) monkfish or cod, cubed
110 g (4 oz) peeled prawns

In a bowl, mix together the honey, soya sauce, tomato purée, vinegar, cornflour and water. Heat the oil in a non-stick frying pan, and stir-fry the onions and peppers for 3 minutes.

Add the monkfish and stir-fry for a further 3 minutes.

Add the prawns and the sauce, and stir again for 2 more minutes.

Variation

• Add a chunk of ginger for a zestier flavour, or add a clove of crushed garlic or garlic purée.

MOTIVATION MATTERS

Tick which of the following reasons for sticking to your diet apply to you. Read through them and think about them often while you slim. Picture yourself in each situation. It will really help to motivate you.

- ❑ I know I will look much better when I'm slim.
- ❑ I will be able to get into all the clothes in my wardrobe.
- ❑ I will be able to buy some new clothes in a smaller size.
- ❑ I will not be ashamed to wear a swimsuit, shorts or a minidress.
- ❑ I may take up a new sport or pastime such as swimming.
- ❑ I will have more confidence to talk to people.
- ❑ I may apply for a new job.
- ❑ I may apply for promotion.
- ❑ I will have the confidence to join a new club or evening class.
- ❑ I will enjoy an improved sex life.
- ❑ My partner will be as pleased as I am when I am slim.
- ❑ My children will be pleased when I am slim.
- ❑ I will be fitter and healthier at the end of my slimming campaign.
- ❑ I will look and feel younger.

CHICKEN DISHES

CHICKEN AND BROCCOLI IN YELLOW BEAN SAUCE

(SERVES 2 AT 270 CALORIES PER PORTION)

1 tbsp corn oil
1 medium onion, finely chopped
1 yellow pepper, de-seeded and sliced
2 small chicken breasts, boned, skinned and sliced
100 g (3½ oz) button mushrooms, sliced
175 g (6 oz) broccoli, cut into small florets
2 tbsp yellow bean sauce
50 ml (2 fl oz) chicken stock from cube
Little salt

Heat the oil in a non-stick frying pan, and stir-fry the onion for 2 minutes. Add the yellow pepper and stir-fry for a further 2 minutes.

Remove the onion and pepper with a slotted spoon, add chicken to pan and stir-fry on High for 3 minutes, until golden.

Return onion and pepper to pan, along with mushrooms, broccoli, sauce and stock. Season to taste and stir-fry for about 4 minutes on a slightly lower heat, until chicken is cooked through. Add more chicken stock, if necessary, and serve.

LEMON CHICKEN STIR-FRY

(SERVES 2 AT 315 CALORIES PER PORTION)

275 g (10 oz) chicken breast fillet, sliced
Juice of half a large, ripe lemon
75 g (3 oz) mangetout *or* French beans, halved
1 medium courgette, cut into thin strips
50 g (2 oz) green pepper, de-seeded and cut into strips
100 ml (3½ fl oz) chicken stock from cube
1½ tbsp dry sherry
1 tbsp soya sauce
1 tsp brown sugar
2 level tsp cornflour
2 tsp corn oil
15 g (½ oz) toasted, flaked almonds

In a bowl, toss the chicken in half the lemon juice; cover and leave for 1 hour, if possible.

Heat the oil in a non-stick frying pan, and stir-fry the chicken for 3 minutes.

Add the mangetout, courgette, pepper and a little chicken stock, and stir-fry for a further 3 minutes, so the vegetables remain crunchy.

Combine the remaining chicken stock with the cornflour, sherry, soya sauce and sugar, and add to pan. Stir-fry for 1 minute.

Toss in the almonds and remaining lemon juice, and serve.

CHILLI CHICKEN WITH AROMATIC RICE

(SERVES 2 AT 400 CALORIES PER PORTION)

2 chicken breast portions, boned and skinned
2 limes (juice of one; one cut in wedges)
1 clove garlic, crushed
Pinch of thyme
1 level tsp chilli powder (or to taste)
Little salt and black pepper
1 tbsp corn oil
1 small onion, finely chopped
100 g (3½ oz) button mushrooms, sliced
75 g (3 oz) [dry weight] long-grain rice
275 ml (10 fl oz) chicken stock from cube

Mix the lime juice with the garlic, thyme, chilli and seasoning, and toss the chicken breast in this mixture. Leave for 1 hour, if possible, turning once.

Brush the base of a shallow ovenproof dish with some of the oil; mix the onion and mushrooms with the dry rice, and spread this mixture on the base of the dish.

Heat the remaining oil in a non-stick pan, and fry the chicken for a few minutes until golden; place on the rice mixture.

Mix the remaining lime juice marinade with heated chicken stock, and pour over the rice and chicken. Bake at 400°F (200°C, Gas mark 6) for approximately 50 minutes. The chicken should be cooked through, all the stock absorbed, and the rice tender.

Serve with lime wedges.

CARIBBEAN CHICKEN

(SERVES 2 AT 225 CALORIES PER PORTION)

50 g (2 oz) desiccated coconut
200 ml (7 fl oz) boiling water
2 chicken breasts, boned and skinned
100 g (3½ oz) pineapple pieces (fresh or in natural juice, drained)
2 tsp cornflour
2 tomatoes, tinned, or skinned and chopped
1 tsp mild curry powder
Pinch All Spice
½ tsp brown sugar
1 tsp tomato purée
1 small red pepper, de-seeded and chopped

Soak the coconut in the boiling water for half an hour.

Cut each chicken breast into 3 or 4 pieces and place in an ovenproof casserole with the pineapple, tomatoes, tomato puree, pepper, spices and sugar.

Strain the coconut milk from the coconut, add the cornflour and stir well. Add to casserole and stir constantly while bringing to a simmer. Place in oven and bake at 350°F (180°C, Gas mark 4) for 50 minutes, or until chicken and vegetables are tender.

TANGY GRILLED CHICKEN

(SERVES 2 AT 210 CALORIES PER PORTION)

2 125g (4½ oz) chicken breast fillets, skinned
2 tsp runny honey
2 tsp wine vinegar
2 tsp olive oil
2 tbsp orange juice
¼ tsp ground ginger
1 level tsp garlic purée
Little salt and black pepper

Slash each breast twice. Combine the remaining ingredients in a bowl, then pour over the chicken and toss to coat.

Leave for 1 hour, if possible, turning once.

Grill the chicken breasts under a medium heat for approximately 20 minutes, basting frequently with the marinade.

Serve garnished with orange slices.

THAI CHICKEN

(SERVES 2 AT 305 CALORIES PER PORTION)

2 tbsp satay marinade
1 heaped tbsp tomato purée
1 tbsp crunchy peanut butter
Dash soya sauce
225 g (8 oz) chicken breast fillets, skinned and cubed
2 tsp corn oil
1 stick celery, finely chopped
4 spring onions, chopped
1 tsp garlic purée

In a bowl, mix together the satay marinade, tomato purée, peanut butter and soya sauce, and add the chicken. Coat thoroughly.

Heat the oil in a non-stick pan and stir-fry the celery and onion for a minute, then add the marinaded chicken pieces and fry over a medium heat for 5 minutes or until they are cooked through, stirring all the time. Stir in the garlic purée. Cook for another 2 minutes, and serve.

CHICKEN BROCHETTES

(SERVES 2 AT 210 CALORIES PER PORTION)

275 g (10 oz) chicken breast fillet, skinned and cubed
1 tbsp olive oil
Juice of half a lemon
2 sprigs fresh or 1 tsp dried thyme
Little salt and pepper
1 bunch watercress, trimmed, washed and patted dry

Place the chicken in a shallow bowl and drizzle with half the olive oil and half the lemon juice. Sprinkle on the thyme, and a little salt and black pepper.

Toss and leave for 1 hour, if possible. Thread the chicken on two skewers, and grill or barbecue for 6 to 8 minutes, turning at least once and basting with any remaining marinade.

Meanwhile, arrange the watercress on two serving dishes. Mix together remaining olive oil, lemon juice and some seasoning, and sprinkle over the watercress. Lay the brochettes on the watercress to serve.

NUTTY CHICKEN WITH BEANSPROUTS

(SERVES 2 AT 285 CALORIES PER PORTION)

175 g (6 oz) chicken breast, boned, skinned and thinly sliced
Half an egg white
1 tsp cornflour
Little salt
1 tbsp corn oil
50 g (2 oz) red pepper, de-seeded and thinly sliced
25 g (1 oz) cashew nuts
1 tbsp dry sherry
1 tbsp soya sauce
100 g (3½ oz) mixed sprouts (e.g., beansprouts, alfalfa sprouts)
50 ml (2 fl oz) chicken stock from cube

Combine the chicken with the egg white, cornflour and salt.

Heat oil in non-stick frying pan and stir-fry the chicken and pepper for 3 minutes. Add the nuts and try for a further minute.

Stir in the remaining ingredients, and fry for a further minute, adding chicken stock as necessary.

> Try to cut down on the amount of salt you add to your recipes. Eating too much salt can lead to fluid retention, especially around the stomach area. Try using a salt substitute such as Lo Salt, or experiment with new herbs and spices to give your recipes added flavour and interest. Buy fresh herbs in preference to dried ones, or grow your own. Freshly cut herbs can be stored inside plastic bags in the fridge.

BEEF, PORK & LAMB DISHES

SAVOURY MINCED BEEF

(SERVES 2 AT 220 CALORIES PER PORTION)

2 tsp corn oil
1 medium onion, very finely chopped
225 g (8 oz) extra-lean minced beef
1 stick celery, finely chopped
1 small carrot, finely chopped
2 tsp tomato purée
1 level tsp mixed herbs
150 ml (5½ fl oz) beef stock, from granules
1 tsp Worcestershire sauce
Little salt and black pepper

Heat the oil in a non-stick frying pan and sauté the onion until transparent. Add the beef and brown, stirring constantly.

Stir in vegetables and remaining ingredients, and simmer for 30 minutes – or until beef and vegetables are tender. Taste for seasoning.

Variation

• For vegetarians, use 225 g (8 oz) TVP mince (reconstituted according to manufacturer's instructions) instead of the minced beef. similarly, use 150 ml (5 ½ fl oz) vegetable stock in place of the beef stock.

CHILLI PEPPERS

(SERVES 2 AT 235 CALORIES PER PORTION)

1 quantity Chilli Con Carne (see recipe, page 69)
2 medium red or green peppers, de-seeded and halved lengthways
4 tbsp low-fat natural yoghurt
Pinch Paprika

Blanch the peppers for a few minutes in boiling, salted water; drain and pat dry. Place peppers in a baking dish and fill each half with the chilli mixture.

Cover the dish with foil and bake at 350°F (180°C, Gas mark 4) for approximately 40 minutes or until peppers are tender.

To serve, top each pepper half with 1 tbsp yoghurt and a sprinkling of paprika.

Variation

• Fill peppers with Bolognese sauce or Meat-free Bolognese Sauce (see recipe, page 58). This would make the calorie content 250 a portion.

CHILLI CON CARNE

(SERVES 2 AT 195 CALORIES PER PORTION)

- 1/2 quantity Savoury Minced Beef (see recipe, page 68)
- 150 g (5 1/2 oz) canned red kidney beans, drained and rinsed
- 1 small red or green pepper, de-seeded and chopped
- 2 tbsp Passata (Italian sieved tomatoes), or chopped, canned tomatoes
- 1 level tsp chilli powder (or to taste)

Mix together all ingredients and simmer for 20 minutes, or until red or green pepper is tender. Taste for seasoning, and adjust accordingly.

Variation

• You can make a type of Chiilli Con Carne suitable for vegetarians by using TVP mince instead of Savoury minced Beef (see recipe variation, page 68).

PORK AND PINEAPPLE STIR-FRY

(SERVES 2 AT 290 CALORIES PER PORTION)

- 225 g (8 oz) lean pork fillet, cut into strips
- 1 tbsp corn oil
- 6 spring onions, halved
- 1 medium red pepper, de-seeded and sliced
- 4 rings fresh or canned pineapple
- 150 g (5 1/2 oz) beansprouts
- 1 tbsp soya sauce
- 1 level tsp stir-fry seasoning (available from supermarkets)

Heat the oil in a non-stick frying pan and stir-fry the pork on high until it is golden.

Turn down the heat, add the onions and peppers, and stir-fry for a further 3 minutes.

Add the pineapple, beansprouts, soya sauce and seasoning, and stir-fry for 1 minute.

For a moister stir-fry, add a little chicken stock at the end of cooking time and allow to bubble.

Variation

• Carrots or courgettes can be added to this dish.
• Tofu or Quorn are suitable pork substitutes for vegetarians.

LAMB BURGERS

(MAKES 2 BURGERS AT 220 CALORIES EACH)

- 175 g (6 oz) minced, lean lamb
- 15 g (1/2 oz) chopped hazelnuts
- 25 g (1 oz) wholemeal breadcrumbs
- half medium egg, beaten
- 2 tsp tomato purée
- 1 small onion, very finely chopped
- Little salt and black pepper
- Pinch dried thyme

Thoroughly blend together all ingredients in a bowl and form into 2 burgers. Grill or dry-fry for 10 minutes, turning once.

REMEMBER

Vary your meal choices as much as possible for maximum nutritional benefit and to prevent the boredom factor from setting in. Get into the habit of planning your meals well in advance to minimise your chances of cheating. Remember, eating plenty of raw foods, vitamin C-rich and spicy foods will help speed up your metabolic rate.

8 The Fat Burning Routine

When most of us say we want to lose *weight*, what we really mean is that we want to lose *fat*. One way to do this is of course to eat less to create a calorie deficit that forces the body to use its own fat stores for energy – which is what happens when we go on a diet. The other, very important way to lose fat is to 'burn it off', through exercise and activity.

Activity of all kinds uses up energy (or calories) and so, broadly speaking, every little bit of movement that you make will help your slimming programme. But by far the quickest and most efficient way of burning up your actual body fat is regular *aerobic* exercise. Not only can aerobic exercise burn off the calories that you eat, but it works on those fat stores as well.

Aerobic exercise – as opposed to, say, a stretching routine or a series of body-toning exercises – is exercise that speeds up your heart and pulse rate, as well as increasing the amount of oxygen that your lungs take in. You breathe harder and more deeply.

To be effective, aerobic exercise must be *sustained* – so running up a short flight of stairs isn't actually aerobic, because it doesn't last long enough. It also has to be *steady*; exercises that you can maintain at the same level for many minutes at a time, feeling neither under- or over-exerted.

The most popular forms of aerobic exercise are walking, jogging, cycling and swimming.

The reason aerobic exercise works so well to burn fat and help slim you is that the body needs fuel to maintain a period of such exercise. First, this fuel comes from your store of glycogen, which you will remember is a fluid composed mainly of glucose and water that is stored in the liver and muscles, as an energy reserve. As the muscles gradually exhaust the supply of glycogen, the body's own fat stores are metabolised, with the help of the increased oxygen in the system, into a usable source of energy. Eventually, if you exercise aerobically for long enough (longer than fifteen minutes or so) fat becomes the greater source of fuel, until, at around thirty minutes into the exercise, it is virtually the *only* source of fuel.

And, even better, if you do regular aerobic exercise and gradually get yourself fitter, you will increase your body's ability to burn fat. This is mainly because fitter lungs have greater capacity – and can breathe in more oxygen – and a fitter heart can pump the oxygen-containing blood round your body much more efficiently. So there is more oxygen present to help burn the fat. Remember, you can't burn fat without oxygen.

But aerobic exercise has more benefits than just calorie- and fat-burning:

• *It increases your metabolic rate* during and *after* the period of exercise, which can save you as much as 100 calories a day. It appears that the exercise literally 'stokes you up', to keep your metabolism ticking over at a higher rate for up to twenty-four hours.

• *It makes you fitter*. Of course, we all want to be fit as well as slim, and aerobic exercise is really the only way to improve your cardio-vascular (heart/lung) fitness.

• *It increases your muscle size*. Another word for muscle is 'lean tissue', and if you exercise regularly the proportion of lean tissue in your body will increase, as the fat decreases. This lean tissue is much more 'metabolically active' than fat, meaning that if you increase your lean tissue bulk, your metabolism will be naturally improved.

• *It provides a better shape.* Virtually everyone who regularly exercises aerobically finds that their shape improves, particularly in the lower body – legs, hips and stomach. Increased muscle tone obviously gives you a better shape, but it also seems that stubborn fat deposits on hips, bottom, stomach and thighs can be shifted through regular aerobic exercise. If you consider that your body is literally 'melting off' its own fat when you do heat-producing aerobic exercise, it's not really surprising, is it?

• *It improves your well-being.* Regular aerobic exercise can make you feel better: livelier and happier, with fewer minor ailments, a greater sense of relaxation and an enhanced ability to cope with life. This is probably partly due to the increased oxygen uptake, partly to the increased metabolic rate and partly to the release of adrenalin that gives you a 'natural high'.

So *do* make time for this aerobic fat-burning programme. It could change not only your shape and your size – but your life, as well!

FITNESS ASSESSMENT

Before you start exercising aerobically, we need to find out how fit, or unfit, you are. We can do this by taking three separate pulse measurements – your resting pulse rate (RPR), exercise pulse rate (EPR), and recovery pulse rate (RPR). Your pulse rate is the rate at which your heart beats.

First, it will be necessary to answer some simple questions, for your own safety. All exercise must be carried out at a level right for you. Attempt a programme that is too difficult, and the results could be disastrous. Second, in order to burn calories and fat efficiently while you exercise aerobically, we need to know whether or not you are working at an aerobic rate – and the pulse tests will tell us this.

What you will be doing is *low-intensity* aerobic exercise, which is aerobic exercise that makes your heart work at between sixty and seventy per cent of its maximum capability.

Your potential maximum is calculated by deducting your age from 220. For example, if you're 30, your maximum rate is 190 beats per minute. To work at low-intensity aerobic levels, then, your heart would need to beat between 114 and 133 beats per minute (sixty to seventy per cent of 190 beats).

If your heart is beating *slower* than this, then the exercise you are doing is *not* aerobic and you need to work *harder*. If your heart is beating *faster* than this, then the work you are doing is approaching high-intensity aerobics, which are more strenuous. As a rule of thumb, up to eighty-five per cent of your maximum heart rate is considered to be within the safe aerobic training zone; however in the early stages of a fitness/slimming campaign you would not be able to sustain exercise at this level for long before becoming tired/breathless/achy, at which point you should stop. This, of course, will quickly bring down your pulse rate, so nothing is gained from going higher than the seventy per cent level.

YOUR FITNESS ANALYSIS

Answer the following questions, ticking the appropriate boxes.

Are you age fifty or over?	Yes ☐	No ☐
Have you been very inactive for five or more years?	Yes ☐	No ☐
Do you have a Body Mass Index (BMI) of 30 or over (see pages 21–22)?	Yes ☐	No ☐
Have you been ill recently, or are you ill now?	Yes ☐	No ☐
Are you pregnant, or have you given birth within the last three months?	Yes ☐	No ☐
Have you any physical complaint that has made exercise difficult in the past (e.g., backache, arthritis)?	Yes ☐	No ☐

If you have answered *yes* to *any* of the above questions then you should have a full consultation with your doctor, to discuss the advisability of beginning this (or any other) exercise programme.

If you receive permission to begin you *must* start the programme on Level 1, Standard 1, no matter what your resting pulse rate tests say.

Taking Your Pulse

Place the first and second finger of your right hand on the pulse spot just below your left jawline, about halfway between your chin and ear. Don't press too hard. Using a watch with a second hand, count the beats. Count for ten full seconds – or for one minute, as instructed in the following tests. Don't measure your pulse with your thumb; it has its own pulse beat. You can also measure your pulse rate in your inner wrist, but the neck beat is usually stronger and much easier to locate.

Test 1: Resting Pulse Rate

After a period of inactivity, take your pulse (as described above) for a full minute. Write down your result here:

My resting pulse rate (RPR) on

.... (date)

is .... (beats per minute).

Check your result against the list below. Come back in a month's time and check your RPR again; if you have been undertaking the fat-burning programme, you will be fitter and your RPR should be lower.

MEN	WOMEN	
70 or under	75 or under	Excellent
71 – 85	76 – 90	Average
86 or over	91 or over	Poor

NB: Pulse rates vary enormously so this is nothing more than an indication of your level of fitness. It is possible to have a slow pulse rate and still be unfit.

My result is ....

Test 2: Exercise Pulse Rate

Now we need to find out whether your pulse rate will stay at a reasonable (though aerobic) level during a fairly typical session of aerobic exercise. Your exercise pulse rate (EPR) relates to your level of fitness: the more unfit you are, the more beats per minute your heart will make to provide your body with the oxygen it needs to do that exercise. A strong, fit heart is a heart that can pump *more* blood and oxygen round your body in a single beat: consequently it beats more slowly as you become fit.

So, when you perform the following step test, you can expect one of three results:

• If you are fitter than average, your heart will be so capable of coping with the test that your pulse rate won't even go as high as the sixty per cent of your maximum required for the exercise to be aerobic. That will mean you are fitter than average and need to work *harder* to get benefits.

• If you are about average fitness, your pulse rate will be within the sixty and seventy per cent of maximum range that we're looking for. The test will be providing you with an aerobic workout.

• If your pulse rises much higher than sixty or seventy per cent, you are not as fit as you could be; in other words, you will find the step test hard. If you are unable to complete the test, or if your pulse rises above the safe upper limit of eighty-five per cent of your maximum, you are probably very unfit, and need to do less demanding exercise until your fitness level improves.

The Step Test

For the test you will need a step, a stair or a sturdy platform of around eight inches (20 cm) high, plus a watch or timer with a second hand. Wear training shoes and comfortable exercise clothing, and warm up by walking on the spot for 1 minute.

• Now, stand in front of the step, and step on and off it (up and down) for 3 minutes. Step up with your right foot; then bring your left up. Put your left foot back on the floor, then bring your right foot down. This movement comprises *1 step*. Do approximately *20 steps* per minute, or *60 steps* in all.

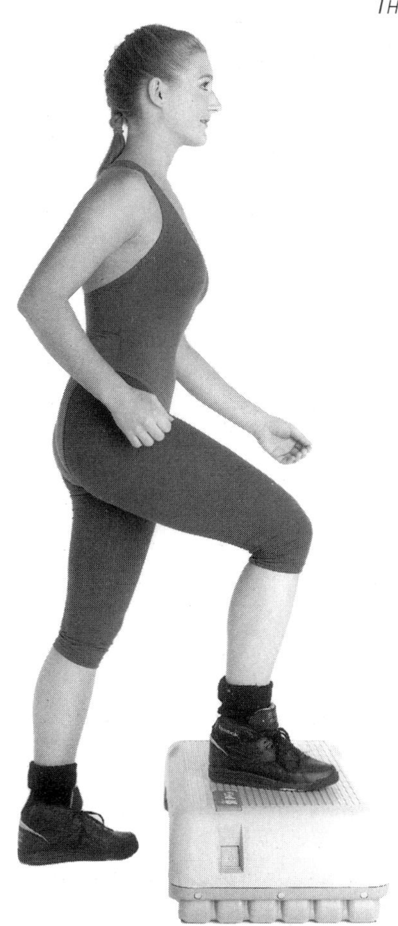

Change the leading foot if you like, but try not to lose the rhythm.

• *As soon as* you finish the test, take your pulse (as explained above) for *10 seconds*. Record the answer below.

> My exercise pulse rate (EPR) on
>
> .... (date) is
>
> .... (beats per ten seconds)

• Using your age (or the nearest to it) and your EPR, look on the chart below to find out the band in which your heart rate was working during the step test. For example, if you are 30 and your EPR is approximately 23 beats per 10 seconds, your Percentage Heart Rate is just over 70 per cent, which is fine. Check the chart immediately below to see what your result means.

Under 60 %	Excellent
60 – 70 %	Good
71 – 85 %	Fair to poor
Over 85%	Very poor
(or unable to complete the test)	

PERCENTAGE HEART RATE CHART

	60%		70%		85%		MAXIMUM BEATS PER MINUTE
AGE	10 SECS	1 MIN	10 SECS	1 MIN	10 SECS	1 MIN	
20	20	120	23	140	28	170	200
25	19.5	117	22.5	136	27.5	166	195
30	19	114	22	133	27	161	190
35	18.5	111	21.5	129	26	157	185
40	18	108	21	126	25.5	153	180
45	17.5	105	20.5	122	25	149	175
50	17	102	20	119	24	144	170
55	16.5	99	19	115	23	140	165
60	16	96	18.5	112	22.5	136	160
65	15.5	93	18	108	22	132	155
70	15	90	17.5	105	21	127	150

NB: When measuring your pulse rate during a workout, it is more accurate to measure for 10 seconds (and either read off the 10-second result, or multiply by 6 to read off the 1-minute result) than it is to *count* the beats for a full minute. During the course of a minute, your heart rate will slow down considerably, giving a false reading.

Test 3: Recovery Pulse Rate

This tests the rate at which you recover from aerobic work; obviously, the quicker your pulse rate returns to normal, the fitter you are likely to be.

This test involves doing the same step test as in Test 2 (see page 72).

• Carry out the step test. Wait one full minute after completion (time this minute on your watch or timer).

• Now take your pulse for 10 seconds (as described above).

The result is .... beats per 10 seconds.

• Multiply this figure by 6.

The result is .... beats per minute.

This is your Recovery Pulse Rate. Check the following details to see what your result means.

MEN	WOMEN	
Pulse less than 70	Pulse less than 78	Excellent
70 – 80	79 – 85	Very good
81 – 90	86 – 94	Average
91 – 100	95 – 109	Poor
Over 100	Over 110	Very poor

Write your results (very good, average, etc.) for all three tests here:

TEST 1: resting pulse rate (RPR)

my rating was ....

TEST 2: exercise pulse rate (EPR)

my rating was ....

TEST 3: recovery pulse rate (RPR)

my rating was ....

The following guidelines will tell you how to begin your aerobic fat-burning programme.

• If you rated all *excellents*, or a mixture of *excellents* and *very goods*, you can start the programme on Level 2, Standard 4.

• If you rated all *very goods*, or a mixture of *very goods* and *averages/fairs*, start on Level 1, Standard 1, but bear in mind that you may progress more quickly than average.

• If you rated all *poors* or *very poors*, start on Level 1, Standard 1, but bear in mind that your fitness level is probably not good and you should take your time.

THE PROGRAMMES

On any level, you have a choice of regular *walking* or regular *cycling*. You will simply work through your chosen programme, moving on to the next Standard as soon as your *exercise pulse rate* drops below the sixty to seventy per cent low-intensity bracket.

This system of levels and standards allows you to move through the exercises at your own pace. As long as you maintain an EPR of between sixty to seventy per cent throughout the programme, you will improve your fitness, and burn fat.

How it works

Begin on the level and standard suggested above. Test your pulse halfway through the exercise period by timing it for ten seconds, immediately after pausing the routine.

Commit the figures for your ten-second sixty to seventy per cent heart rate to memory (see chart, page 73). For instance, if you are aged thirty you will know that for the work you are doing to be low-intensity aerobic, your ten-second pulse count should be between nineteen and twenty-two. Lower than that and the standard you are on isn't giving you enough work. In this case, move up a standard.

If your pulse count is higher than that, the standard is working you harder than necessary. If the pulse count is only one or two figures above your ideal, say, in the case of the a thirty year old, twenty-three or twenty-four, you may stay on that standard. Over the days you'll see your pulse rate come down.

If your pulse rate is way over, say, near the eighty-five per cent level, the work is probably too hard for you, and you should move back a level.

Stay on any given standard until your pulse count drops *below* the sixty per cent level. Then move up a standard.

Fill out the programme charts as you go along. Write down the date you start and finish each level and standard, and record your comments.

Frequency

You may do the programme as often as you like for up to six days a week. Bear in mind that the more often you do it, the more calories you will expend, the more fat you will burn, and the higher you will raise your metabolic rate.

Therefore, if you are a Low Met (see pages 23–24), I suggest you try to do the programme six times a week for maximum benefit. If you are an Average Met, four or five times a week should be sufficient. If you are a High Met, aim to do the programme at least three times a week.

Instructions

Here are some instructions that will apply whether you choose to do the *walking* or the *cycling* programme:

• Build up the pace of your workout by doing the first two minutes out at a steady pace. This also acts as a warm-up. Similarly, ease off the pace of the last two minutes in order to cool down.

• Wear suitable clothes. If the weather is cold, it is better to wear several thin layers that you can peel off as you warm up. Take a cycle bag or rucksack to put these clothes in. Also take a low-calorie drink in case you get thirsty, especially on the longer sessions.

• Check pulse rate at least once during the session – more if you like. Adjust the pace according to the results.

• If for any reason you can't time your pulse rate, (for instance if you forget to take your watch with you), you can use the *perceived effort* test to ascertain whether the work you are doing is aerobic. This isn't as accurate as a true pulse measurement, but it is a surprisingly good guide. And if you have been doing aerobic exercise for more than a few days you will begin to be able to tell when you are working between sixty and seventy per cent.

The perceived effort test

1 – very very light 2 – very light 3 – light 4 – fairly light	Warm-up stage equivalent
5 – moderate 6 – somewhat hard 7 – hard	60 – 70 % equivalent
8 – very hard 9 – very very hard	85 % + equivalent

Another simple way to test whether your exercise is aerobic is the talking/breathing test. During low-intensity aerobic work you should be breathing more heavily than usual, but at a rate which allows you to talk. If you are unable to speak, you're working too hard.

If you are warm, breathing deeply and moving steadily, your action should be aerobic. If you have to stop and regain your breath at all during your workout, you are working too hard. *Remember:* to burn fat, your body needs oxygen. If you are working so hard that your heart/lung system can't keep up with the necessary oxygen supply (which is what breathlessness is) then the work you are doing is not aerobic.

You also risk fatigue and possibly more serious problems if you work too hard, so never work until you're gasping for breath.

• The programme assumes that you'll be walking or cycling on flat land, so if you live in hilly country, take into consideration the fact that working uphill will be harder and downhill easier. At the beginning of the programme, do try to work on level ground.

• The ideal programme is one where you measure the distance you travel on each outing. For this, you will need either a cycle milometer or a pedometer (or you could measure out the distance beforehand in a car). If none of these methods is possible, you can follow the alternative time-based walking

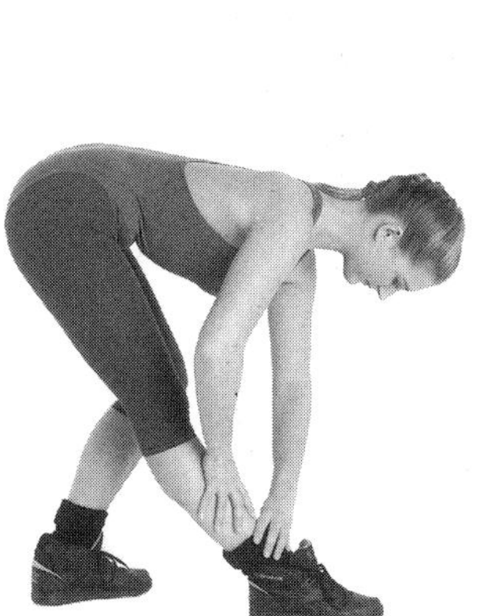
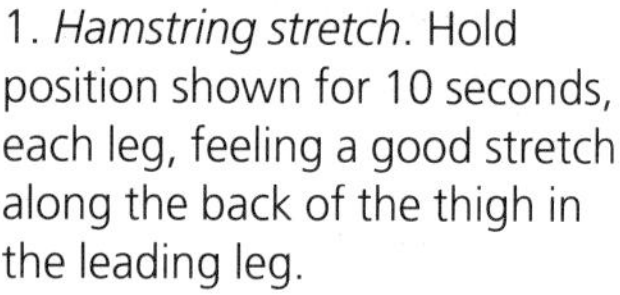
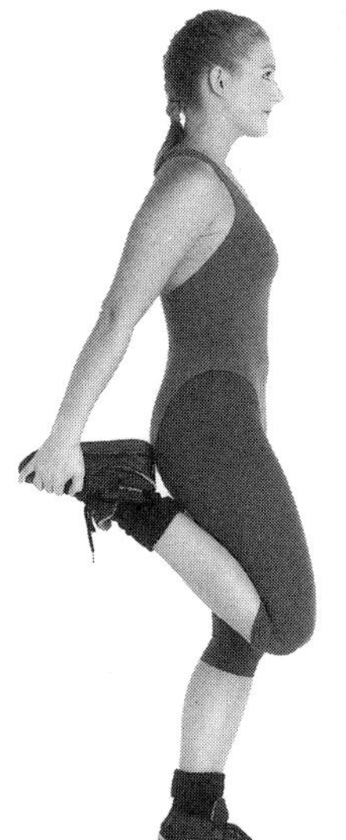
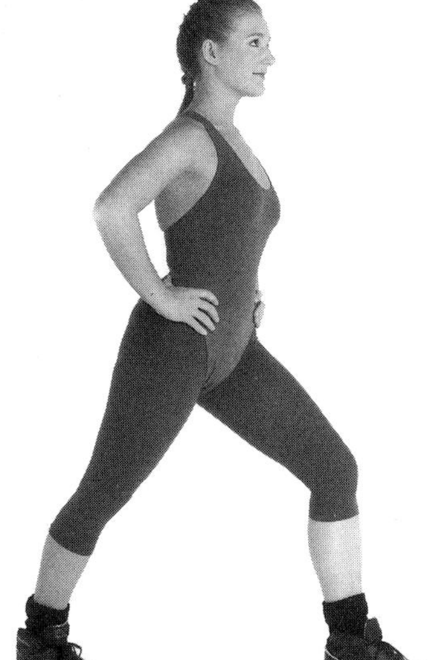
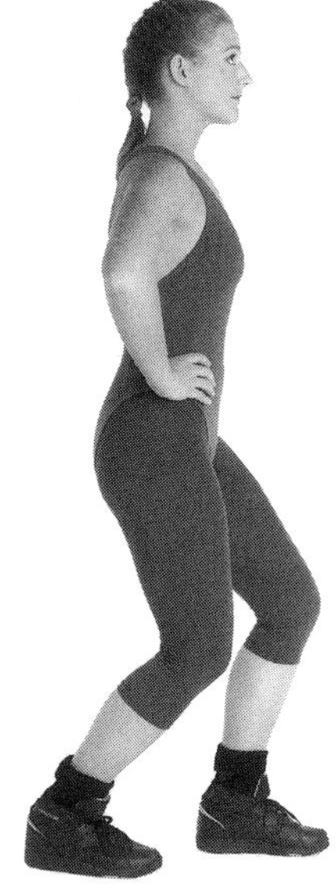

1. *Hamstring stretch.* Hold position shown for 10 seconds, each leg, feeling a good stretch along the back of the thigh in the leading leg.

2. *Quad stretch.* Hold position shown for 10 seconds, each leg.

3. *Calf stretch.* Stand as shown, feeling a good stretch in upper calf on the back leg. Hold for 10 seconds, each side.

4. *Lower calf stretch.* Stand as shown, feeling a good stretch around lower calf and back of ankle. Hold for 10 seconds, each side.

programmes, based on time alone rather than distance and time.
• After each session, do some leg stretching exercises (as above) to help prevent any stiffness.

Safety

Don't walk or cycle alone in remote areas or deserted city areas, particularly after dark and particularly if you are female. Try to walk or cycle with a friend of the same fitness level as you. Or choose an aerobic alternative (see below).

Occasional Alternatives

You may already be involved in one or more of the following pastimes, each of which, if done in an aerobic manner (steadily and continuously, preferably for at least twenty minutes) can occasionally be done instead of the walking or cycling routine.

However, look on these as occasional alternatives, for it is impossible to give you a graded programme for them here. The exceptions are that you can use an indoor treadmill instead of outdoor walking, or an exercise cycle instead of outdoor cycling, as long as both have distance/speed gauges. You might like to try the following:

• Swim (bearing in mind that it is not easy to swim continuously in most public pools because they are so busy);
• Attend an aerobics class or exercise to an aerobics video;
• Attend a step class or exercise to a step video;
• Roller skate;
• Dance;
• Row on a machine or in a boat.

Cycling

Special instructions

• Before you begin, check your cycle for safety – brakes, tyres, rusty bolts, lights, bell, etc.
• If you haven't cycled in a long time, make sure you start in a very quiet area, ideally off-road.
• Buy a cycle helmet and use it.
• If you rated very unfit on the fitness tests, you may be wise to walk for the first week or two of your programme. When you feel a bit fitter, change to cycling.

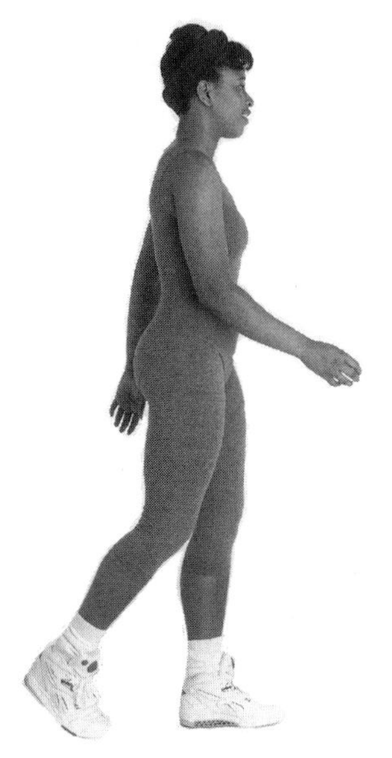

1. *Warm-up walking.* Use for first and last 2 minutes. Take even strides, arms lightly swinging.

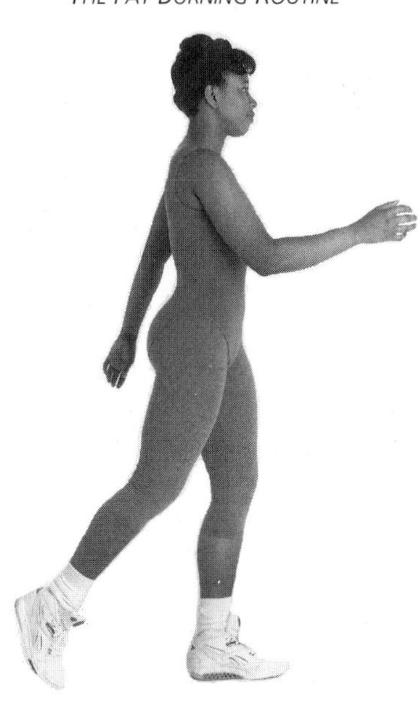

2. *Brisk walking.* Use for most of your walk. Longer strides from the hip; arms pumping higher.

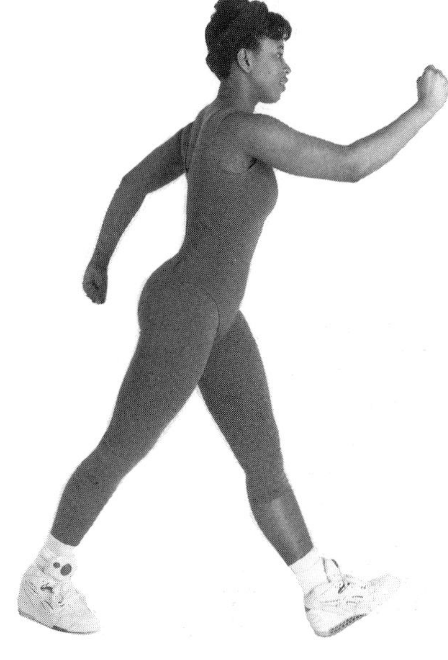

3. *Very brisk walking.* Use as you get fitter. Arms pump really high, stride extended and flowing. Wrist and ankle weights can also be worn when you are even fitter.

• Use as high a gear as you can for the work involved.

Walking

Special instructions

• Walk with your stomach and bottom tucked in, using long rhythmic strides.
• Wear comfortable cushioned walking shoes. Walking is a low-impact aerobic exercise, unlike running, but even so, it pays to give your feet support and comfort. Be very fussy about fit and comfort when buying a pair of shoes for fitness walking.

WARNING: If while exercising you feel nauseous, dizzy, faint, or undue discomfort or pain of any kind, *stop* and get help. When carrying out this or any exercise programme it is vital that you comply with the instructions given for maximum safety. If you still experience any physical problem, you *must* seek your doctor's advice immediately.

Be More Active

As we discussed earlier, every little activity that you do helps to burn off calories, so try to build more activity into your life. Here are some ideas of how you can do that. Fill in some of your own.

- Take the stairs instead of a lift or escalator whenever possible.
- Run up the stairs instead of walking.
- Leave the car at home and walk whenever possible.
- Always attempt to walk briskly instead of dawdling.
- Enjoy more active sports such as dancing, hiking, tennis and golf.
- Cut down the amount of television you watch and use that time to do something more active.
- Stand rather than sit whenever you can.

My ideas:

- ....
- ....

WALKING PROGRAMME

Throughout this programme, my exercise pulse rate should remain

between .... (beats per 10 secs [60%]) and .... (beats per 10 secs [70%])

LEVEL 1

	DISTANCE/TIME PROGRAMME	TIME PROGRAMME	PROGRESS MONITOR
Standard 1	Walk 1 mile (1.6 km). Take 30 minutes. Walking pace: 2 miles per hour (mph) (3.2 kph). Check your pulse.	Walk 15 mins out. Take note of point reached. Walk back. Walking pace: moderate/ comfortable. Check your pulse.	Date started Standard 1: .... Date finished Standard 1: .... Total days spent on Standard 1: .... Comments: ....
Standard 2	Walk $1^1/_4$ miles (2 km). Take 30 minutes. Walking pace: $2^1/_2$ mph (4 kph) Check your pulse.	Walk 15 mins out, same route as Standard 1. Walk as far past point reached in Standard 1 as you can (within the 15 mins). Take note of new point reached. Walk back. Walking pace: comfortable. Check your pulse.	Date started Standard 2: .... Date finished Standard 2: .... Total days spent on Standard 2: .... Comments: ....
Standard 3	Walk $1^1/_2$ miles (2.4 km). Take 30 minutes. Walking pace: 3 mph (4.8 kph). Check your pulse.	Walk 15 mins out, same route as Standard 2. Walk as far past point reached in Standard 2 as you can (within the 15 mins). Take note of new point reached. Walk back. Walking pace: as brisk as you can manage within EPR.	Date started Standard 3: .... Date finished Standard 3: .... Total days spent on Standard 3: .... Comments: ....

Remember to choose Distance/Time Programme *or* Time Programme *not* both.

WALKING PROGRAMME

LEVEL 2

	DISTANCE/TIME PROGRAMME	TIME PROGRAMME	PROGRESS MONITOR
Standard 4	Walk 2 miles (3.2 km). Take 40 minutes. Walking pace: 3 mph (4.8 kph). Check your pulse.	Walk 20 mins out (preferably on a new route). Take note of point reached. Walk back. Walking pace: brisk. Check your pulse.	Date started Standard 4: .... Date finished Standard 4: .... Total days spent on Standard 4: .... Comments: ....
Standard 5	Walk 2 1/3 miles (3.7 km). Take 30 minutes. Walking pace: 3 1/2 mph (5.6 kph). Check your pulse.	Walk 20 mins out, same route as Standard 4. Walk as far past point reached in Standard 4 as you can (within the 20 mins). Take note of new point reached. Walk back. Walking pace: brisk. Check your pulse.	Date started Standard 5: .... Date finished Standard 5: .... Total days spent on Standard 5: .... Comments: ....
Standard 6	Walk 2 2/3 miles (4.2 km). Take 40 minutes. Walking pace: 4 mph (6.4 kph). Check your pulse.	Walk 20 mins out, same route as Standard 5. Walk as far past point reached in Standard 5 as you can (within the 20 mins). Take note of new point reached. Walk back. Walking pace: striding. Check your pulse.	Date started Standard 6: .... Date finished Standard 6: .... Total days spent on Standard 6: .... Comments: ....

Remember to choose Distance/Time Programme *or* Time Programme *not* both.

WALKING PROGRAMME

LEVEL 3

	DISTANCE/TIME PROGRAMME	TIME PROGRAMME	PROGRESS MONITOR
Standard 7	Walk 3¼ miles (5.2 km). Take 50 minutes. Walking pace: 4 mph (6.4 kph). Check your pulse.	Walk 25 mins out (preferably on a new route). Take note of point reached. Walk back. Walking pace: striding. Check your pulse.	Date started Standard 7: .... Date finished Standard 7: .... Total days spent on Standard 7: .... Comments: ....
Standard 8	Walk 3¾ miles (6 km). Take 50 minutes. Walking pace: Striding at 4½ mph (7.2 kph). Check your pulse.	Walk 25 mins out, same route as Standard 7. Walk as far past point reached in Standard 7 as you can (within the 25 mins). Take note of new point reached. Walk back. Walking pace: striding. Check your pulse.	Date started Standard 8: .... Date finished Standard 8: .... Total days spent on Standard 8: .... Comments: ....
Standard 9	Walk 5 miles (8 km). Take 1 hour. Walking pace: 5 mph (8 kph). Check your pulse.	Walk 30 mins out, same route as Standard 8. Walk as far past point reached in Standard 8 as you can (within the 30 mins). Walk back. Walking pace: extended stride. Check your pulse.	Date started Standard 9: .... Date finished Standard 9: .... Total days spent on Standard 9: .... Comments: ....

Remember to choose Distance/Time Programme *or* Time Programme *not* both.

Once you have reached Level 3, Standard 9, you can either maintain that level of fitness, or, if you want to improve further, add your own speeds/mileages to walks. You can also add weights to your body for increased effect, or do all uphill work.

CYCLING PROGRAMME

Throughout this programme, my exercise pulse rate should remain

between .... (beats per 10 secs [60%]) and .... (beats per 10 secs [70%])

LEVEL 1

	DISTANCE	TIME	SPEED	PROGRESS MONITOR
Standard 1	1 to 2 miles (1.6 to 3.2 km)	Go at a pace to suit yourself until completely confident. Check pulse twice and keep it within your own EPR (above).		Date started Standard 1: .... Date finished Standard 1: .... Total days spent on Standard 1: .... Comments: ....
Standard 2	2 miles (3.2 km)	15 mins	8 mph (12.8 kph)	Date started Standard 2: .... Date finished Standard 2: .... Total days spent on Standard 2: .... Comments: ....
Standard 3	4 miles (6.4 km)	24 mins	10 mph (16 kph)	Date started Standard 3: .... Date finished Standard 3: .... Total days spent on Standard 3: .... Comments: ....

Remember to check your pulse as often as you can during these sessions, to ensure that the Standard you are currently working on is suitable for you.

CYCLING PROGRAMME

LEVEL 2

	DISTANCE	TIME	SPEED	PROGRESS MONITOR
Standard 4	6 miles (9.6 km)	30 mins	12 mph (19.2 kph)	Date started Standard 4: .... Date finished Standard 4: .... Total days spent on Standard 4: .... Comments: ....
Standard 5	7 miles (11.2 km)	30 mins	14 mph (22.4 kph)	Date started Standard 5: .... Date finished Standard 5: .... Total days spent on Standard 5: .... Comments: ....
Standard 6	8 miles (12.8 km)	30 mins	16 mph (25.6 kph)	Date started Standard 6: .... Date finished Standard 6: .... Total days spent on Standard 6: .... Comments: ....

CYCLING PROGRAMME

LEVEL 3

	DISTANCE	TIME	SPEED	PROGRESS MONITOR
Standard 7	10 miles (16 km)	38 mins	16 mph (25.6 kph)	Date started Standard 7: ...... Date finished Standard 7: ...... Total days spent on Standard 7: ...... Comments: ......
Standard 8	12 miles (19.2 km)	40 mins	18 mph (28.8 kph)	Date started Standard 8: ...... Date finished Standard 8: ...... Total days spent on Standard 8: ...... Comments: ......
Standard 9	15 miles (24 km)	45 mins	20 mph (32 kph)	Date started Standard 9: ...... Date finished Standard 9: ...... Total days spent on Standard 9: ...... Comments: ......

Once you have reached Level 3, Standard 9, you can either maintain that level of fitness, or, if you want to improve further, add your own speeds/mileages to rides. You can also add weights to your body for increased effect, or do all uphill work.

The Body Shaping Routine

9

Dieting and fat-burning aerobic exercise are two sides of the 'slim/fit' triangle, but it is as important not to neglect the third side: body shaping.

If you don't shape your body through strength, tone and flexibility exercises, you are likely to have one – or probably more than one – of the following figure defects: a weak, rounded back; flabby upper arms; a floppy and fat tummy; a thick waist; spreading hips; wobbly thighs; a flat bottom; a dropped rear; baggy knees; and shapeless calves and ankles.

In fact, many people who think they are fat really aren't. These figure faults are just as likely to be due to lack of exercise as to a weight problem.

The good news is that anyone can improve their shape – and improve it quickly. Strength and tone exercises will replace the slack, flabby look with a firm, healthy, rounded and defined shape. A good stretching programme will not only develop flexibility, but will also ensure that your new, firm look is slim and sleek.

In just twelve minutes a day the body shaping routine outlined here combines strength, tone and flexibility exercises to give you that look you've always wanted. There's another reason why you should do the body shaping exercises: a properly exercised body has a *higher* metabolic rate than an unexercised one, because its increased proportion of muscle burns calories faster than fat tissue.

Body Shaping: How It Works

The body shaping system begins with the *basic* routine. This consists of a *warm-up*, 8 *strength/tone* exercises, and a series of *cool-down stretches*. Everyone should do this basic routine; it will give you a complete all-over workout and is suitable for everyone.

Then there are five *supplements:* short routines, each concentrating on a different part of the body. You may do as many of these extra routines as you like. They only take four minutes or so, each. They are:

1 Bust/chest, upper back and arms
2 Waist, stomach and lower back
3 Bottom and hips
4 Thighs and calves
5 Flexibility

To help you decide which supplements you should do – and also to help you discover your current level of strength and flexibility – do the *shape analysis* test below. When you have completed these tests, follow the advice given to decide on your own personal body shaping routine.

SHAPE ANALYSIS

Strength tests

1. Upper body/back

Lie on your stomach with your arms by your sides. Breathe out and raise head and neck off the floor as far as they will go. How far off the floor does your chin go?

Less than 3 ins (7.5 cm)	Poor	☐
3 – 6 ins (7.5 – 15 cm)	Fair	☐
Over 6 ins (15 cm)	Good	☐

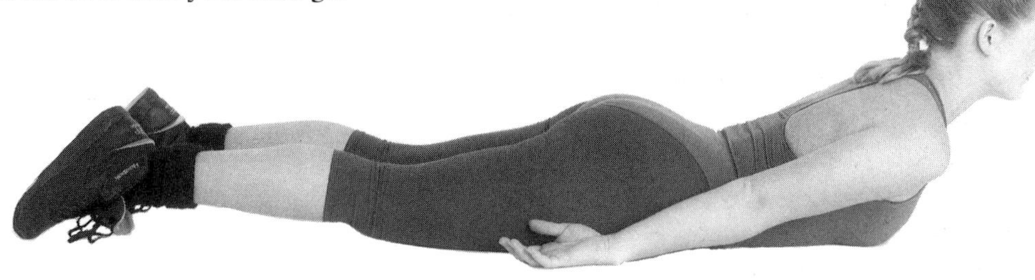

2. Arms

Get in the press-up position (for full instructions, see page 103). How many consecutive press-ups can you do before arm-muscle fatigue (weakness/shaking) sets in?

8 or less	Poor	☐
9 – 20	Fair	☐
Over 20	Good	☐

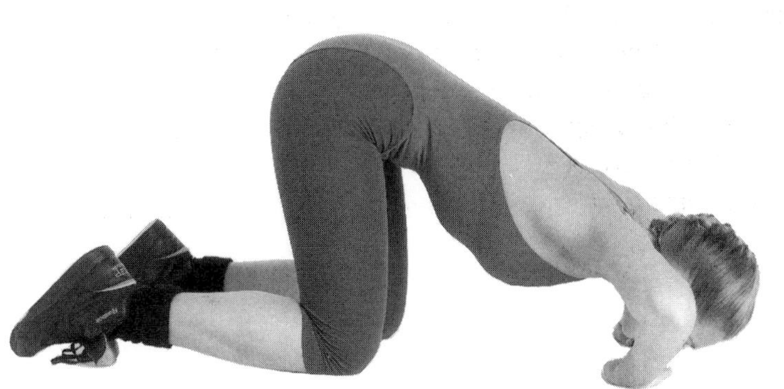

Strength tests (continued) ▶

3. Stomach

Lie on your back with hands at ears, and legs as shown. Keeping legs still, raise head and neck off floor and touch elbow to opposite knee. Return to floor and repeat on other side, keeping elbows back all the time. How many of these diagonal curl-ups can you do (consecutively) before tiring?

8 or less	Poor	☐
9 – 20	Fair	☐
Over 20	Good	☐

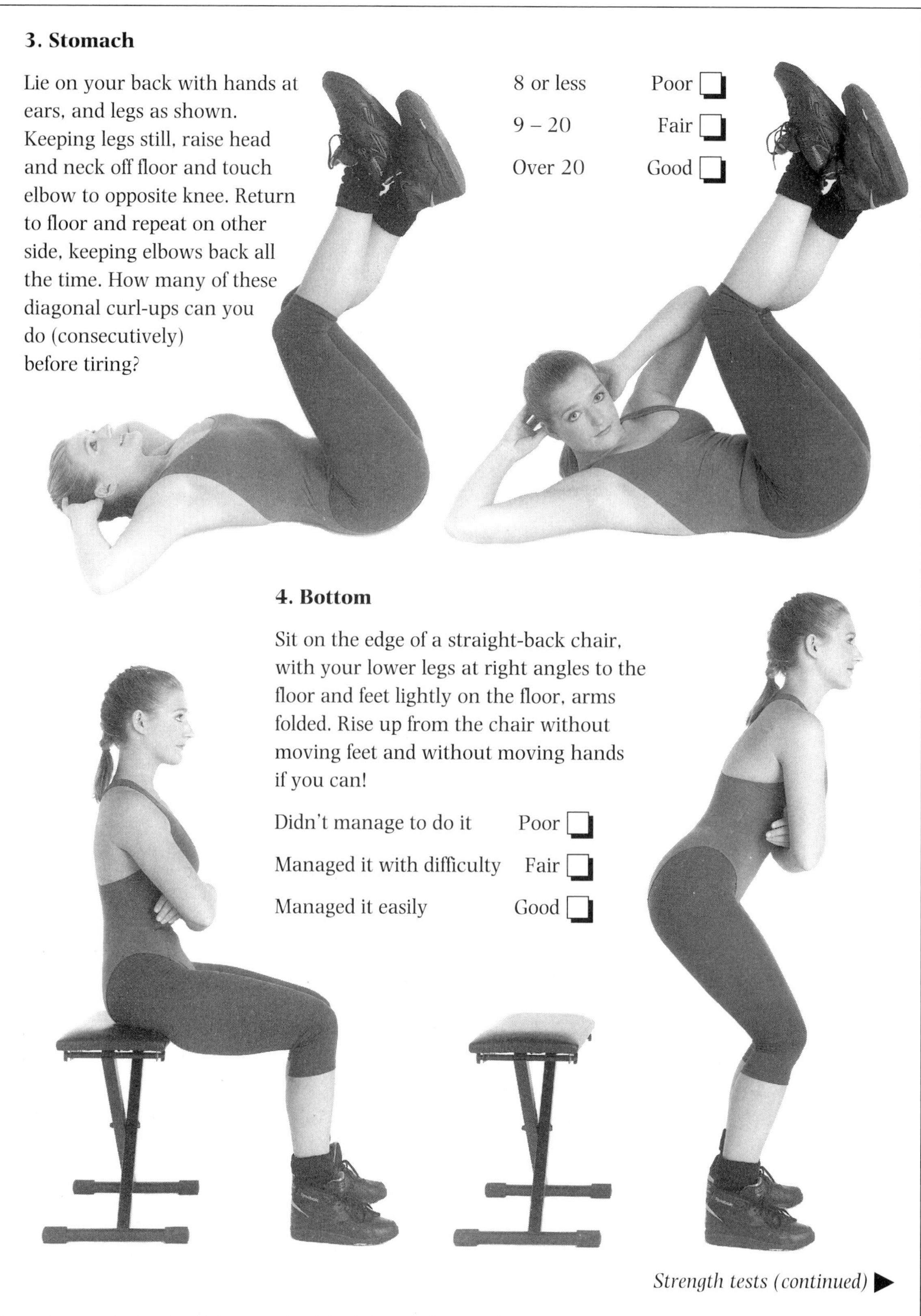

4. Bottom

Sit on the edge of a straight-back chair, with your lower legs at right angles to the floor and feet lightly on the floor, arms folded. Rise up from the chair without moving feet and without moving hands if you can!

Didn't manage to do it	Poor	☐
Managed it with difficulty	Fair	☐
Managed it easily	Good	☐

Strength tests (continued) ▶

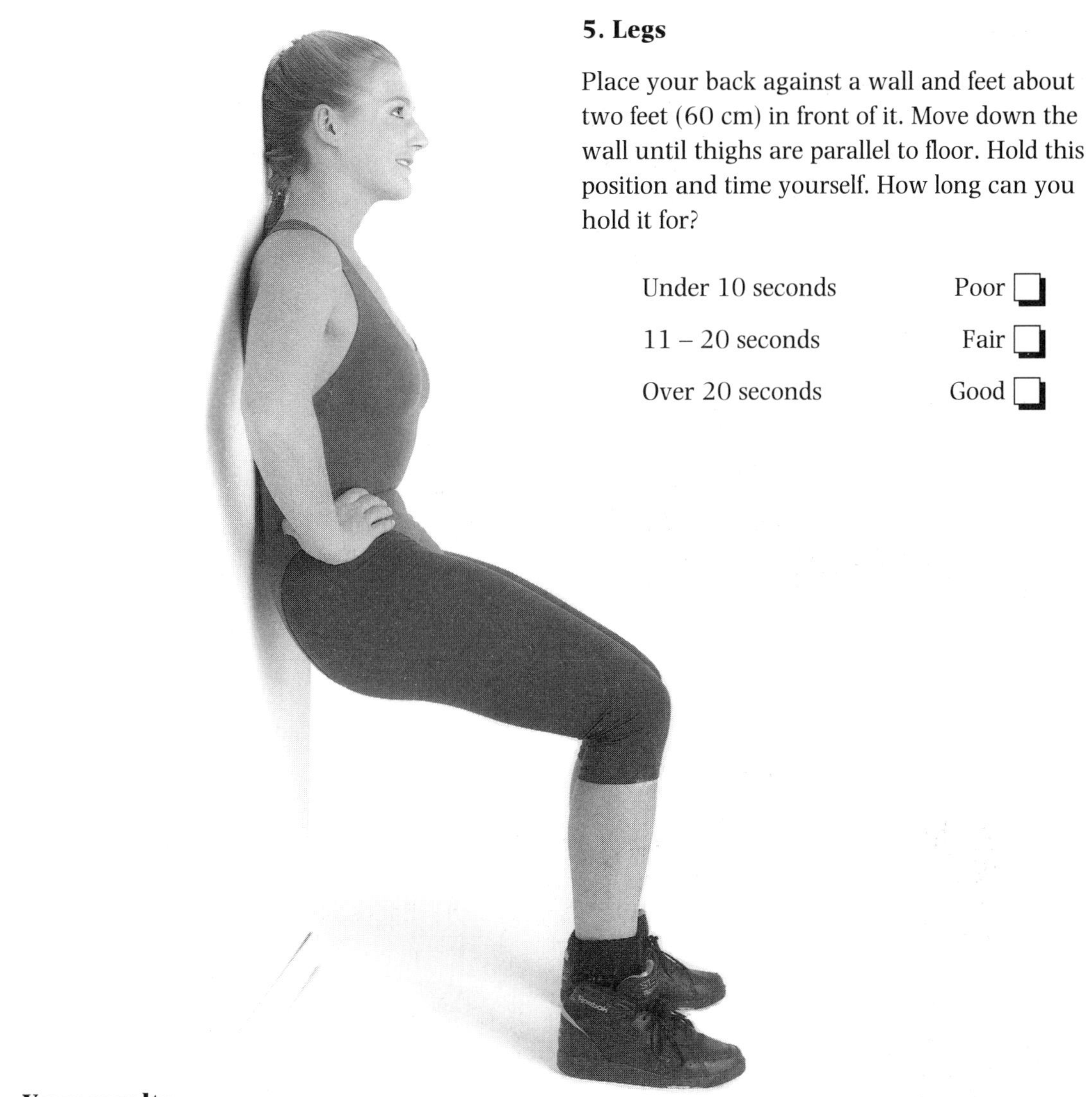

5. Legs

Place your back against a wall and feet about two feet (60 cm) in front of it. Move down the wall until thighs are parallel to floor. Hold this position and time yourself. How long can you hold it for?

Under 10 seconds	Poor ❑
11 – 20 seconds	Fair ❑
Over 20 seconds	Good ❑

Your results

• If you scored *poor* in many of the tests, you can be fairly sure that your strength is poor. Take the *basic* routine at your own pace and you will soon see improvements. When you have been doing this routine for a few weeks, you can add one or more of the supplement routines – perhaps doing one supplement one day, another the next, and so on.

• If you scored *poor* in just one of the tests, you can begin the *basic* routine and add the corresponding supplement routine for your poor result. (For example, if your result in Test 1 [page 85] was poor, you'll need to add Supplement 1 – for upper body.)

• Most people of average fitness will have scored *fair* in many of the tests. You will see rapid improvements if you follow the *basic* routine; improvements will be more rapid if you do extra supplemental work, too.

• If you scored *good* in most or all of the tests, you are of above-average fitness and may start the basic routine with either added weights, or doubling up on sets.

Flexibility tests

1. Shoulders

Stand and place right hand behind neck, arm bent and palm inwards, elbow up as shown. Bring left forearm up behind back as shown, palm outwards. Stretch, without hurting, and try to touch fingers of both hands.

Fingers are inches apart	Poor	❑
Fingers touching or nearly so	Fair	❑
Fingers can link	Good	❑

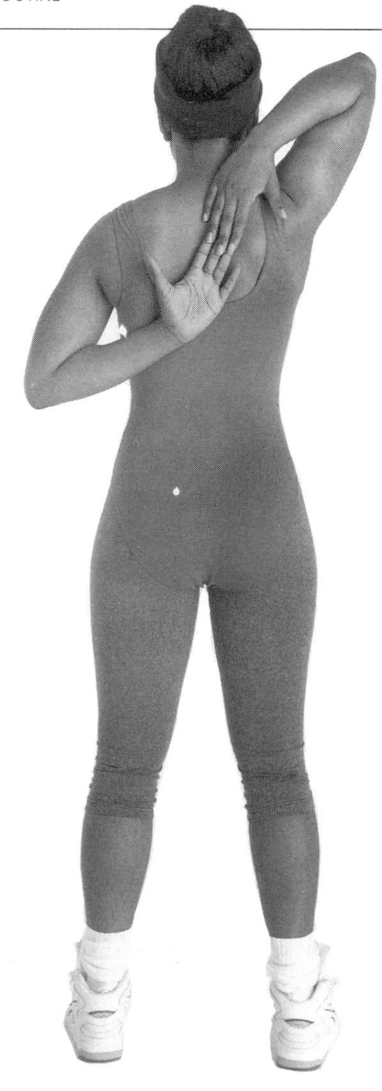

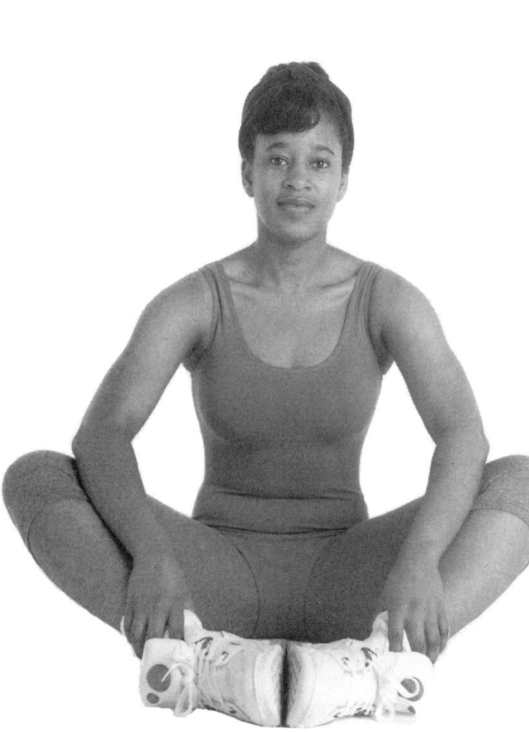

2. Groin

Sit on floor and place feet, soles together, about 9 ins (22.5 cm) in front of groin. Sit up straight. Using elbows and hands to help you as shown, how far towards the floor can your knees reach without pain? (Measure the gap between the lower side of your knee and the floor.)

Over 6 ins (15 cm)	Poor	❑
3- 6 ins (9 – 15 cm)	Fair	❑
Under 3 ins (7.5 cm)	Good	❑

Flexibility tests (continued) 

3. Hamstrings and lower back

Sit with one leg straight out in front of you and the other bent and to the side, as shown. Keeping back straight and *not* curved, lean over the straight leg as far as you can, without feeling pain. When you have leant as far as you can, reach arms out and touch as far down the leg as you can. Don't move back position or hunch over to do this; you must keep lower back strong. How far can you reach?

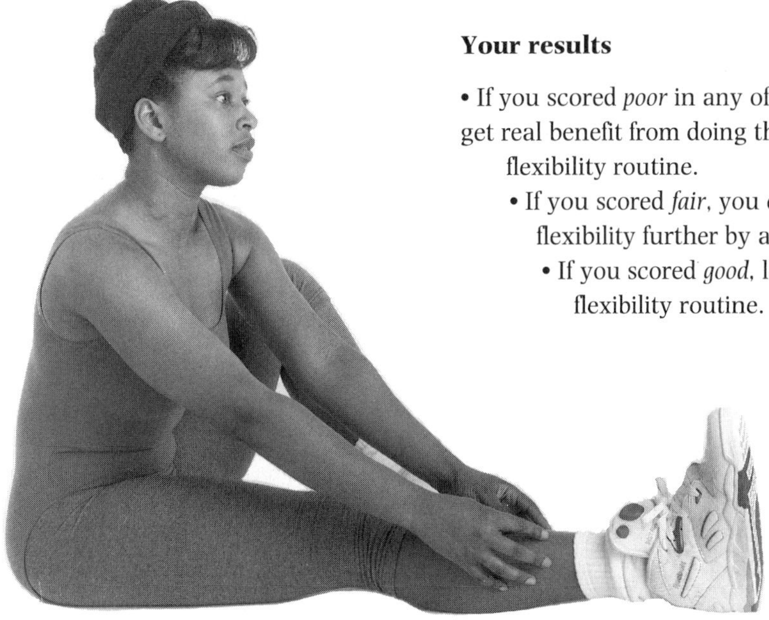

Around knee/calf level	Poor	❑
Around ankle level	Fair	❑
To sole of foot or beyond	Good	❑

Your results

- If you scored *poor* in any of the tests, you will get real benefit from doing the supplementary flexibility routine.
- If you scored *fair*, you can improve your flexibility further by adding the routine.
- If you scored *good*, leave out the flexibility routine.

THE BASIC ROUTINE

The routine consists of a *warm-up*, which should take you a minimum of two minutes, followed by an eight-exercise strength/tone routine, which should take you a minimum of eight minutes. With each exercise there are various tips, and sometimes instructions for an easier, or more difficult version of the exercise. Choose whichever is most applicable to your level of fitness, as gauged by the above tests. Further improvement can be gained by adding ankle and/or wrist weights; you can also add further sets of the repetitions. If you are adding sets, rest ten to twenty seconds between sets.

Take the strength tests again in four weeks' time and then in eight weeks' time and see how much you have improved!

Lastly, there is a *cool-down/stretch* routine. Stretches are best done at the end of a routine while your body is warm; *never* while your muscles are cold. You should hold each stretch for a minimum of ten seconds just at the point where you feel the muscle aching pleasantly. As your body becomes more supple, you can relax into a stretch after the ten seconds and find you can stretch a bit further. Hold this stretch for thirty seconds or more. This will increase your suppleness very effectively. Take the flexibility test in four weeks' time and again in eight weeks' time and see the difference.

How often?

Do the *basics* routine a minimum of three times a week – it only takes about twelve minutes to complete. Even if you are unfit it is important to do the three-times-a-week minimum otherwise you won't see the results. If you like, you can do it up to six times a week.

THE SUPPLEMENTS

Decide which supplements you need to do; in the case of supplements 1–4 do them *after* the *basic* strength routine but *before* the cool-down. If doing supplement 5 you can add it on to the end of the cool down. Each supplement should take no more than four minutes. Alternatively, you could do your supplement on alternate days to the *basics* routine, in which case you must start with a warm-up (same as for basics), and in the case of supplements 1–4 you should finish with the cool-down stretches.

INSTRUCTIONS APPLICABLE TO ALL EXERCISES

- Exercise in a warm room in suitable, comfortable clothing which offers no restriction of movement and allows you to see what your body is doing.
- Wear jazz or aerobic shoes.
- Exercise on a suitable surface: a wooden floor topped by a non-slip exercise mat, or a carpet with a towel laid on it.
- Don't exercise if you are unwell, or within an hour after a heavy meal.
- Check with your doctor before starting this or any other exercise routine.
- Don't stint on the warm-up; it is vital to get your heart, lungs and muscles warm and limber up before you begin.
- Breathe normally throughout. Generally speaking, you should breathe out on the effort, in as you relax.
- It is more important that you carry out the exercises – maintaining a good body posture – than do lots of repeats. Number of reps given are only guidelines; always stop if your working muscle(s) feel(s) exhausted; or, carry on and do more reps if you don't feel worked at all.
- To improve, you should always work up to the point when your working muscle is tired, but not beyond that point.
- Don't lock your knees or elbows.
- Do the exercises with your total concentration and effort. If you feel pain, stop.

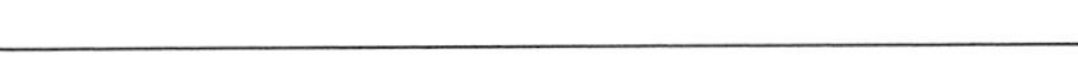

The Warm-up

1. Shoulder circling with toe taps

Stand with legs hip-width apart, knees slightly bent, stomach tucked in. Place hands on shoulders as shown and circle arms and shoulders round, 10 times towards the back, and 10 times towards the front. As you do so, lift toes off floor in time with the circles, keeping heels firmly fixed in their place.

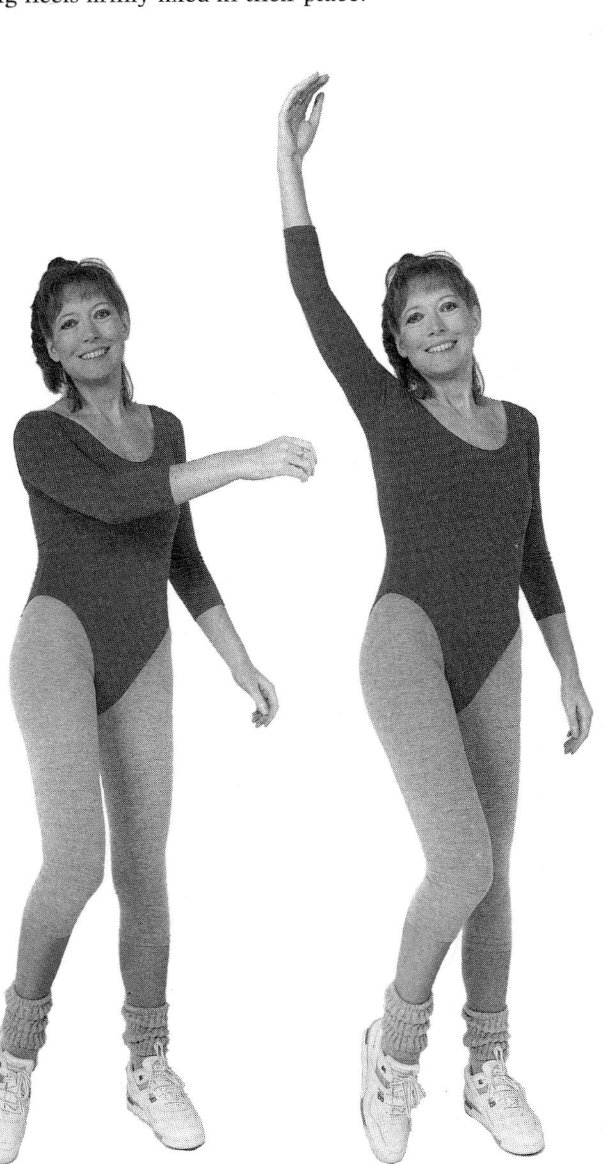

2. Arm circles with leg transfers

Stand with legs 18 ins (45 cm) apart, knees slightly bent. Bring right arm across in front of body, and up and round in a large circle; as you do so, transfer body weight on to left side and bring right leg across. As arm returns to start position, so does right leg. In a flowing movement, left arm makes same circle and left leg moves across. Do 10 arm circles/ leg transfers.

The Warm-up (continued) ▶

3. Spine shake-out

Stand with legs hip-width apart, knees slightly bent and tummy tucked in, hands resting halfway down thighs. Now imagine your spine is a ripple on a pond – smoothly shake it out from top to bottom, tilting your pelvis in and back, and bending your knees a little further to produce the 'rippling' rhythm.

As you go, move your shoulders forward and back, and don't forget to bring your neck forward in line with the top of your spine. It should be fluid, not rigid. Shake out your spine for 30 seconds.

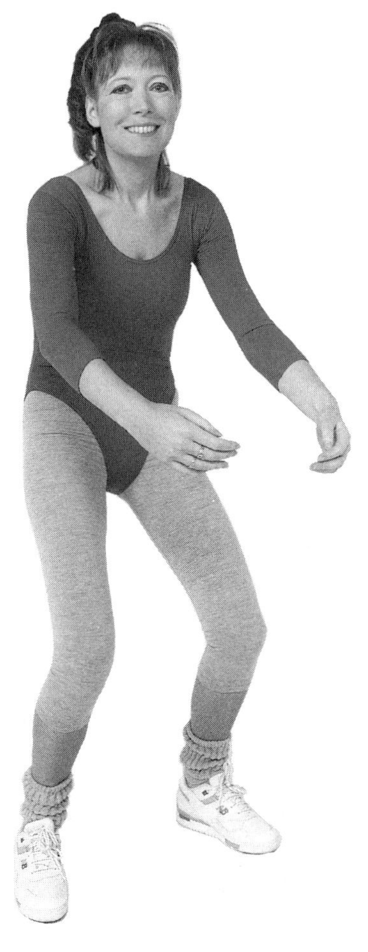

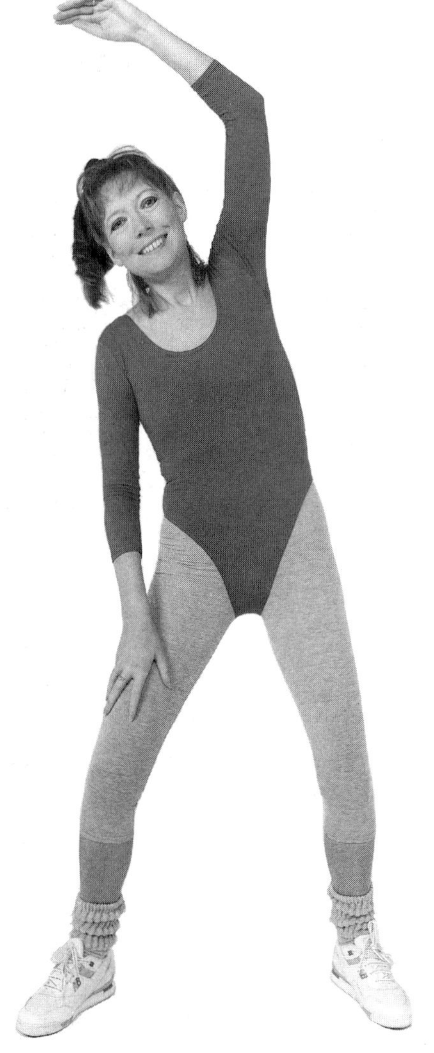

4. Sideways bends

Stand with legs 18 ins (45 cm) apart, tummy tucked in and knees slightly bent. Place right hand lightly on thigh and as you do so, bend right knee and lift left arm high into the air, leaning slightly over to the right.

Return to start and repeat on left side.

Repeat 10 times each side.

The Warm-up (continued) 

5. Waist twists with arm pumps

Stand with legs hip-width apart, tummy tucked in and knees slightly bent, back nice and straight, arms straight out in front of you and hands making fists.

Now, keeping hips still, bring right arm back, bending elbow, and smoothly twist round to the right as you do so, taking head with you.

Come back to start and repeat on left side.

Repeat 10 times each side.

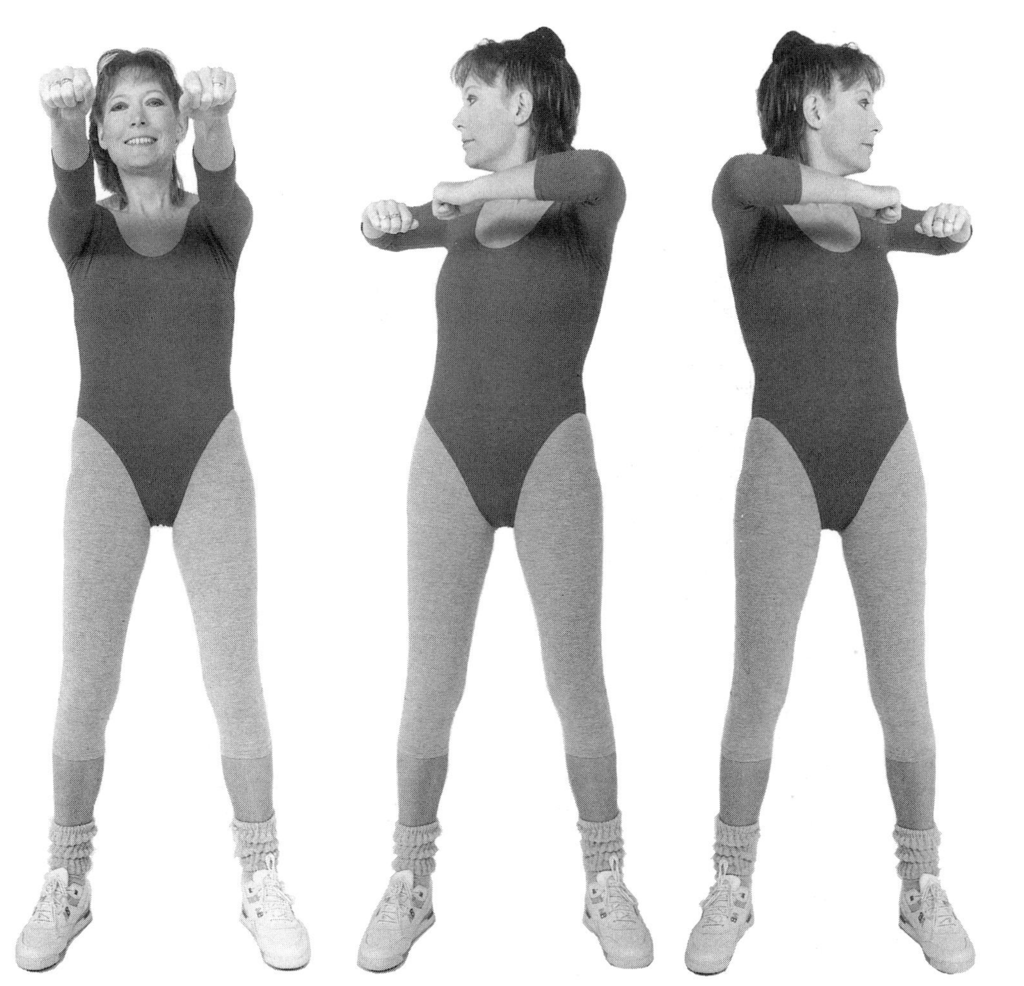

The Warm-up (continued) ▶

6. Puppet on a string

Stand with legs hip-width apart, tummy tucked in and knees slightly bent. Lift arms high above head then bring them down together; as you do so, lift right leg, bent at knee, up between your arms, returning it to the floor as your arms return above head.

Repeat to left side in a rhythmic way.

Repeat for 30 seconds.

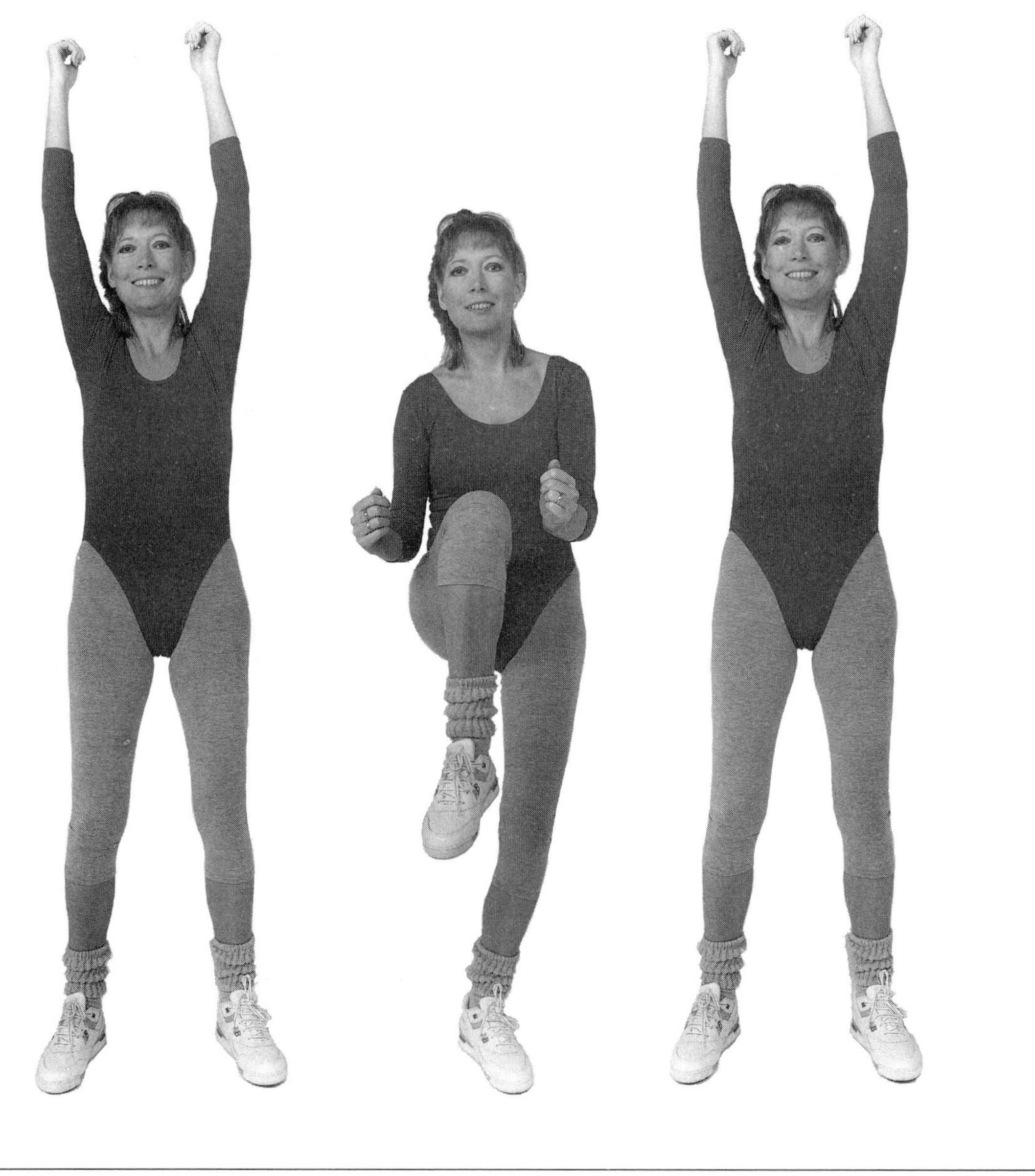

The Routine

1. Squats with elbow presses (for thighs, bottom, arms and chest)

Stand with feet approximately 2 ft (60 cm) apart, knees slightly bent, feet slightly out, tummy tucked in and arms out to sides.

Now bend into a squat, aiming to keep your back straight without leaning forward beyond knees, until your thighs are just above parallel to floor (or as near as you can get).

At the same time, bring your arms round and in, so that forearms meet as shown. Really try to get those elbows touching.

Hold squat for count of one, then return to start.

Repeat 8 times.

- ***Easier***. Do the squats only; try the elbow presses separately. Don't squat so far down. Lean forward.
- ***Harder***. Do additional sets. Make the squats deeper (but don't take thighs below knee level).

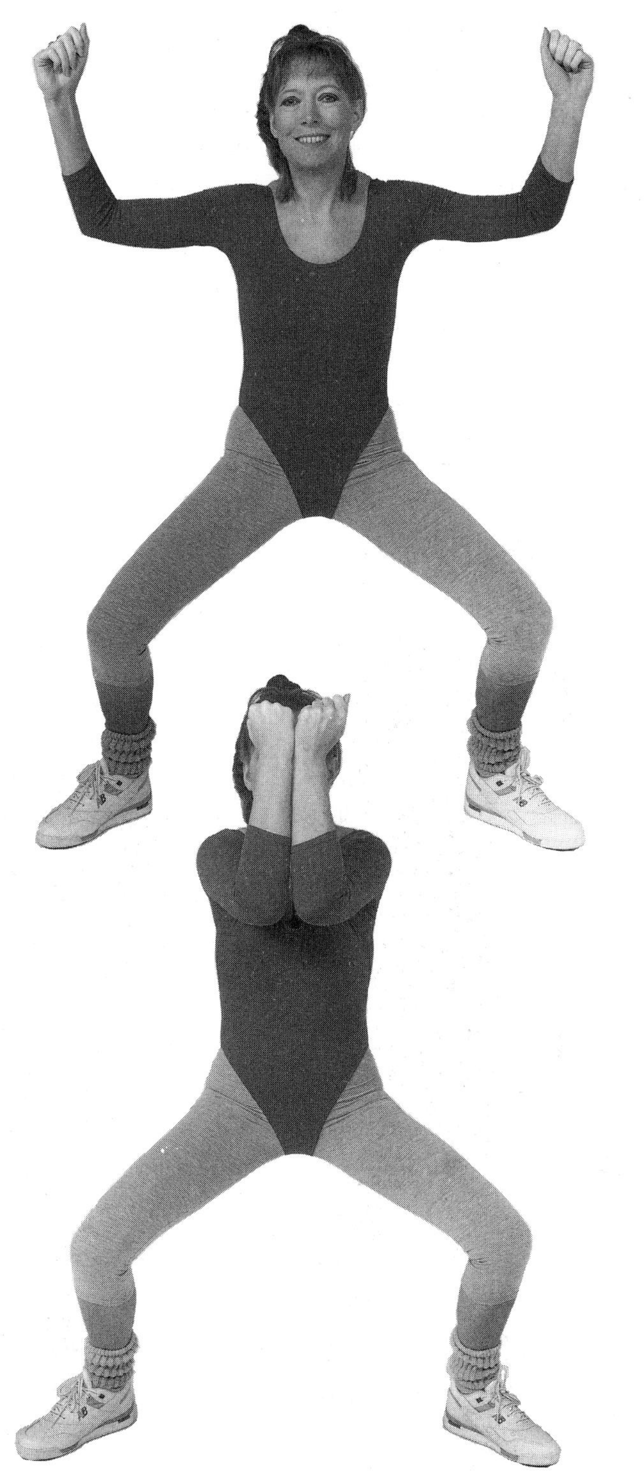

The Routine (continued) ▶

2. Heel raises with shoulder presses (for calves and back)

Stand with feet hip-width apart, tummy tucked in, knees slightly bent, toes facing forward, arms raised to sides as shown. Now lift heels off floor and as you do so, bring arms back to feel muscles around shoulder blades working.

Do 20 heel raises/shoulder presses.

• ***Easier***. Do the heel raises only; try the shoulder presses separately. Don't raise up so high.
• ***Harder***. Do additional sets. Raise higher; squeeze shoulders harder.

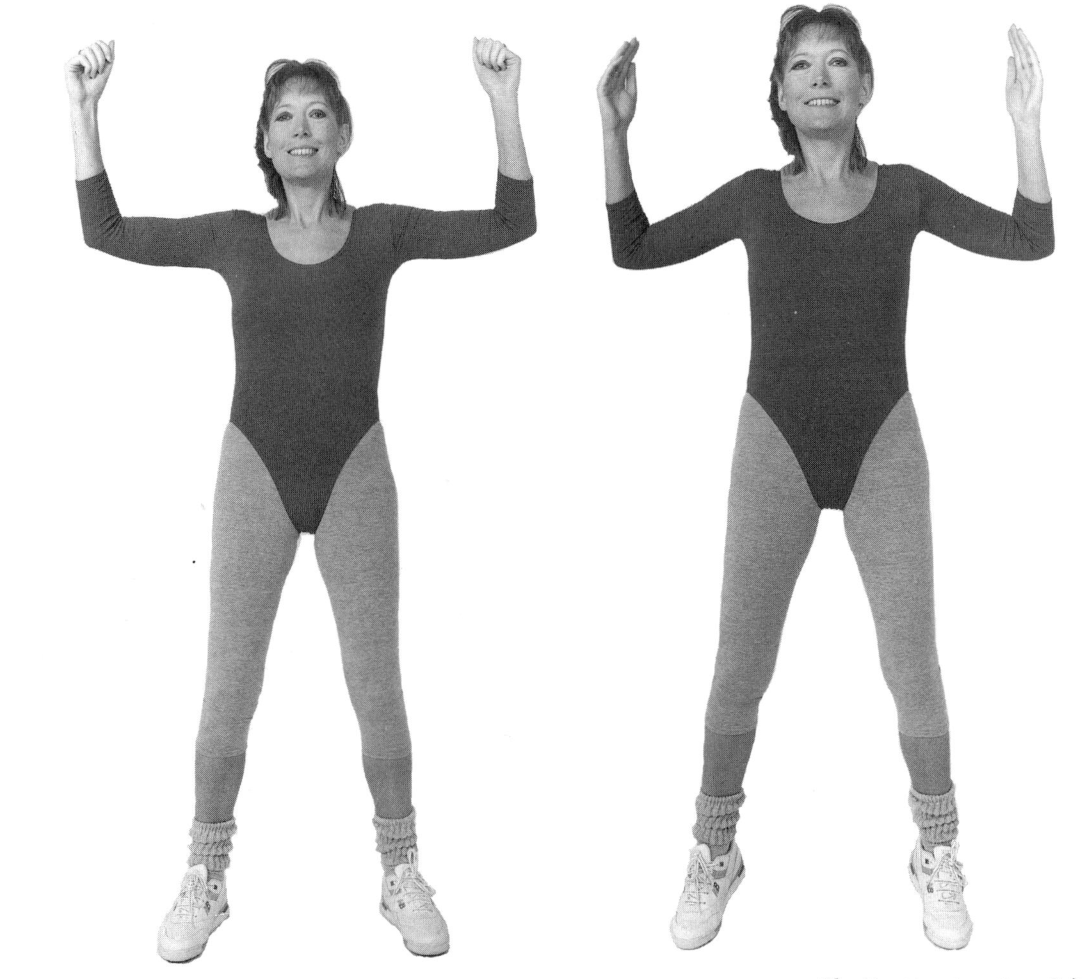

The Routine (continued) ▶

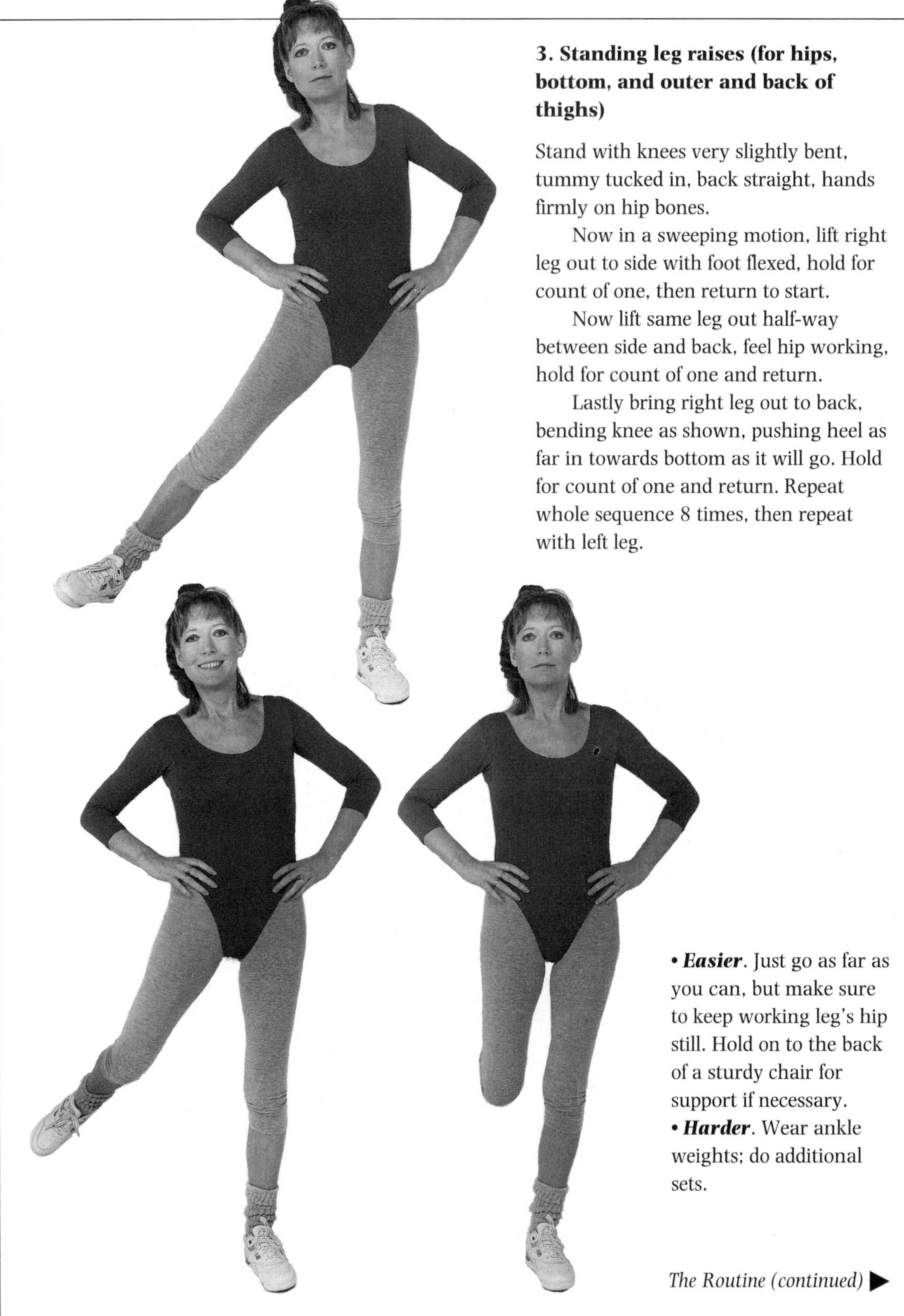

3. Standing leg raises (for hips, bottom, and outer and back of thighs)

Stand with knees very slightly bent, tummy tucked in, back straight, hands firmly on hip bones.

Now in a sweeping motion, lift right leg out to side with foot flexed, hold for count of one, then return to start.

Now lift same leg out half-way between side and back, feel hip working, hold for count of one and return.

Lastly bring right leg out to back, bending knee as shown, pushing heel as far in towards bottom as it will go. Hold for count of one and return. Repeat whole sequence 8 times, then repeat with left leg.

• ***Easier***. Just go as far as you can, but make sure to keep working leg's hip still. Hold on to the back of a sturdy chair for support if necessary.
• ***Harder***. Wear ankle weights; do additional sets.

The Routine (continued) ▶

4. Dips with toe taps (for backs of arms, shoulders, chest and calves)

Sit on mat with knees bent, feet on floor. Place hands on floor just behind either side of back with hands as shown.

Now lower upper body down towards floor. Hold for count of one, slowly raise up again and repeat 8 times.

Throughout the sequence, tap alternate toes lightly on floor.

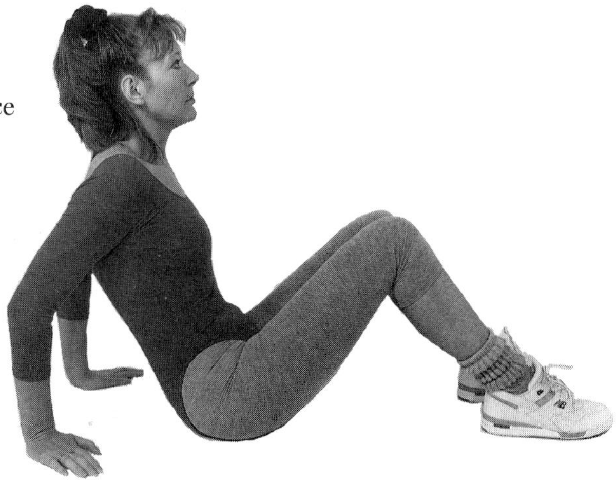

• ***Easier***. The nearer your hands are to your back, the easier the exercise. Omit toe taps to start with, if you like.
• ***Harder***. The further your hands are away from your back, the harder the exercise. You can also start the dips with your body off the floor, supported only with feet and hands, thus dipping down further each time. You can also do additional sets.

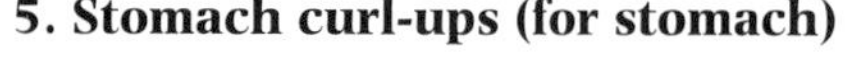

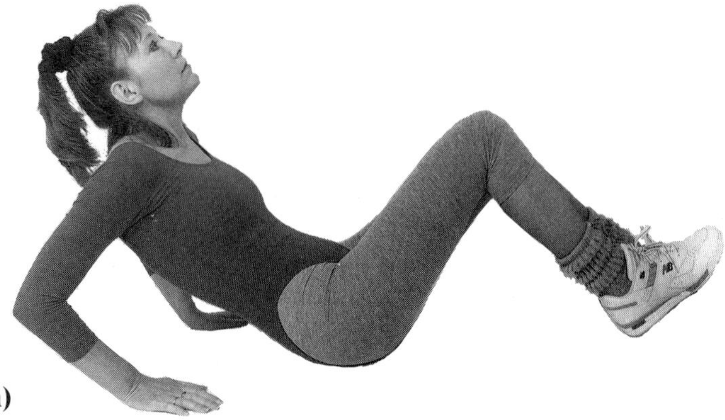

5. Stomach curl-ups (for stomach)

Lie on back on mat with knees bent, feet on floor, hands at ears and elbows out, as shown. Curl head, neck and shoulders off floor, aiming right hand towards left knee.

Hold the furthest you can go for a count of one; slowly return to floor and repeat 8 times.

Change arms and repeat to other side.

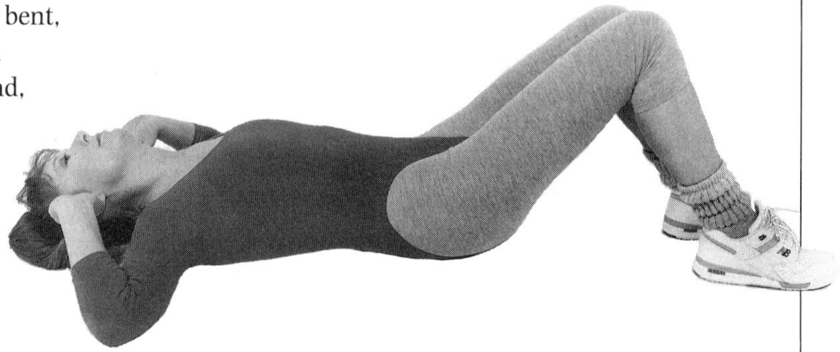

• ***Easier***. Just go as far as you can – the smaller the movement you make off the floor, the easier it is.
• ***Harder***. Hold the 'up' position for a count of two each time; do additional sets.

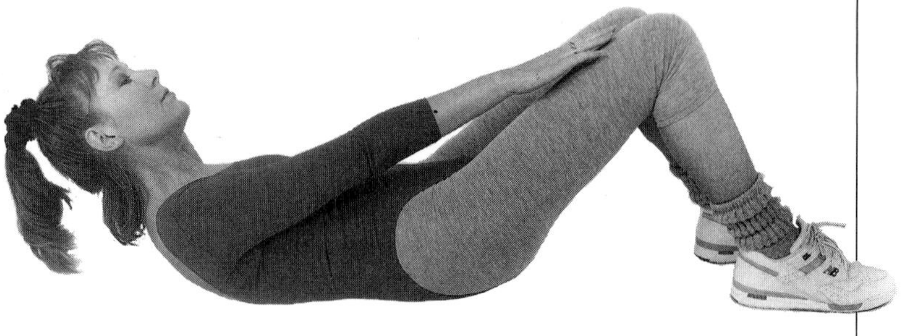

The Routine (continued) ▶

6. Waist curls (for waist and stomach)

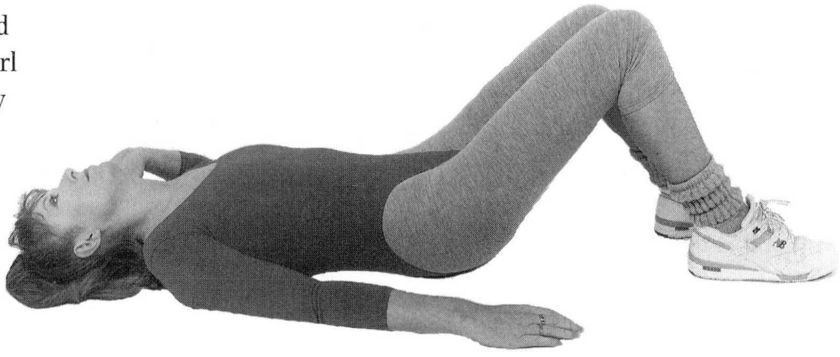

Lie on back as shown. Place left hand just behind left ear and elbow out. Curl head and neck a little way off the floor and this time aim to move shoulders round and down to the right so that your outstretched arm is reaching a point nearer your feet.

Do 8 waist curls to the right, then repeat to the left.

• ***Easier***. Bring right arm up and over body to touch left knee. Repeat 8 times, then repeat to other side.
• ***Harder***. Do additional sets. Do the curls with feet off floor and ankles crossed.

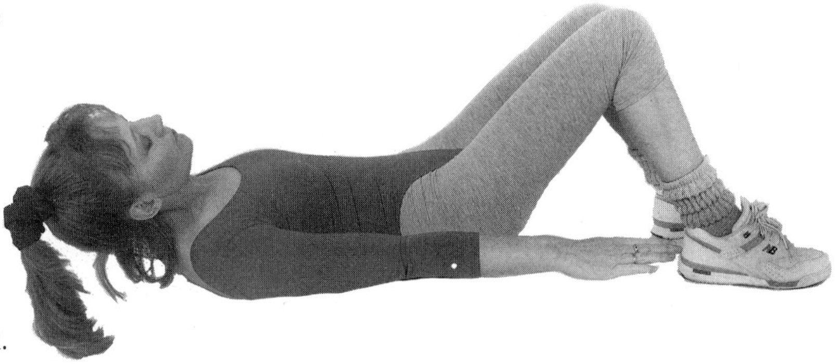

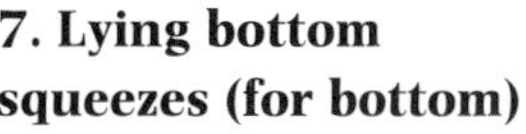

7. Lying bottom squeezes (for bottom)

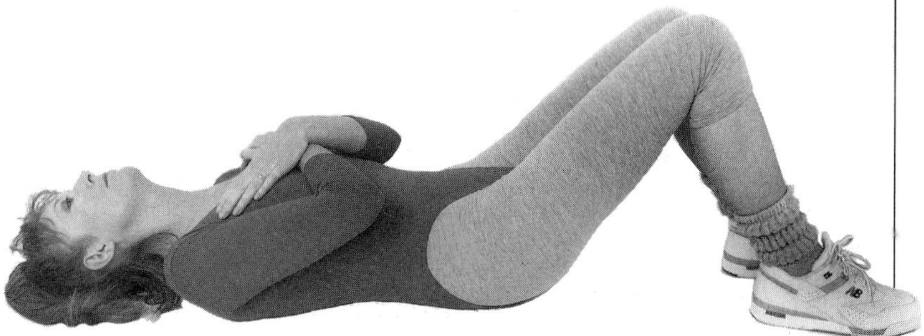

Lie on back with knees bent, feet on floor, hands behind head or crossed on chest. Now using bottom muscles, lift body from shoulders to knees off floor, as shown.

Squeeze bottom tight for a count of two, then slowly return to floor.

Repeat 8 times.

• ***Easier***. Just lift bottom an inch or so off floor at each squeeze.
• ***Harder***. Do additional sets. Do exercise with legs wide apart.

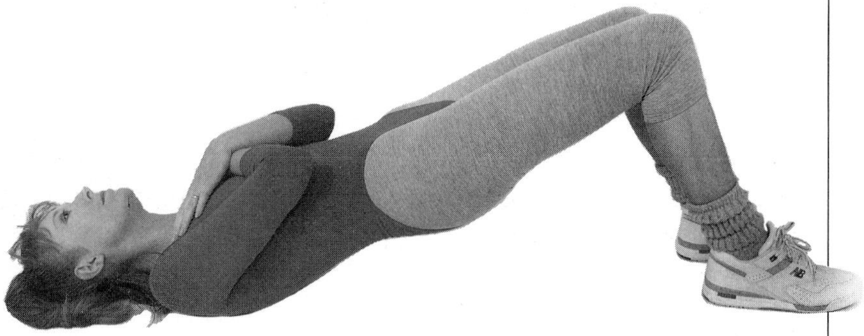

The Routine (continued) ▶

8. Leg and arm raises (for upper and lower back, bottom, backs of thighs and shoulders)

Lie on tummy on floor as shown, with legs straight and right arm stretched out in front. Now, keeping hips relaxed but still on floor, lift right arm and left leg a few inches off floor.

Lower slowly to floor and repeat opposite side.

Do 16 lifts.

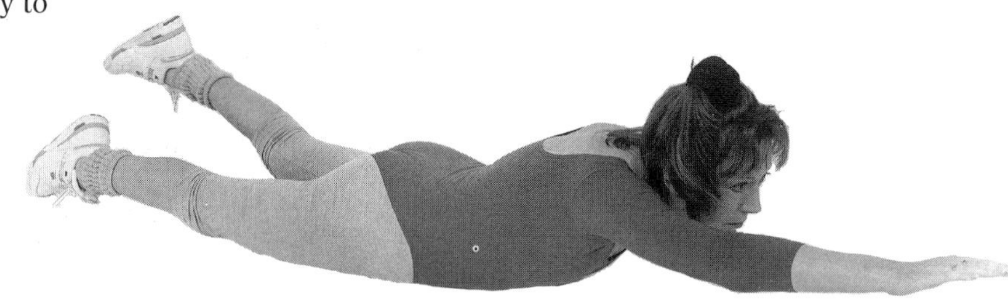

• ***Easier***. Do the arm lifts separately from the leg lifts. Don't try to lift too high.
• ***Harder***. Use wrist and ankle weights. Do additional sets.

Cool-down Stretches

All Stretches should be held for a minimum of 10 seconds, gradually working up to 30 seconds or more.

1. Stomach Stretch

Lying on front, place hands on floor in front of you, as shown, and stretch out stomach and chest.

2. Quad stretch

Lying on tummy, bring right hand round to clasp right foot and bring foot in towards bottom, as shown. Feel the stretch along your front thigh (quad) muscle. Hold for a count of ten, release and repeat with other leg.

As you become more supple you will be able to do this stretch with both legs together.

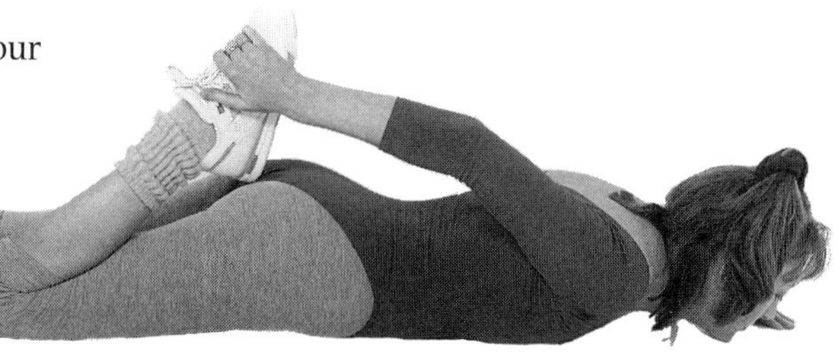

3. Kneeling back and shoulder stretch

Kneel with hands on floor, and arms and back making a straight line. Feel a stretch along back and in shoulders.

For a deeper stretch, move hands a little further along the floor away from knees.

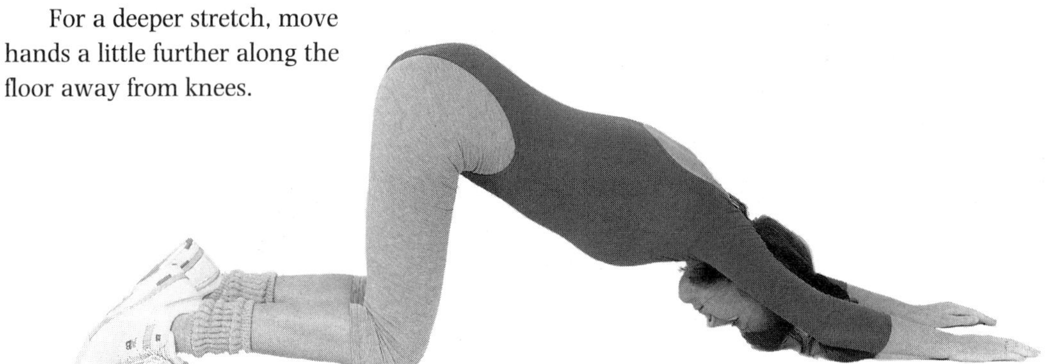

4. Arm stretch

Sit on floor with legs in a comfortable position and back straight. Take right arm up and hand behind centre of shoulders.

Using left hand, clasp right arm just above elbow and slowly pull the right arm back so that your right hand travels further down your back.

Repeat to other side. Feel the stretch along upper arm.

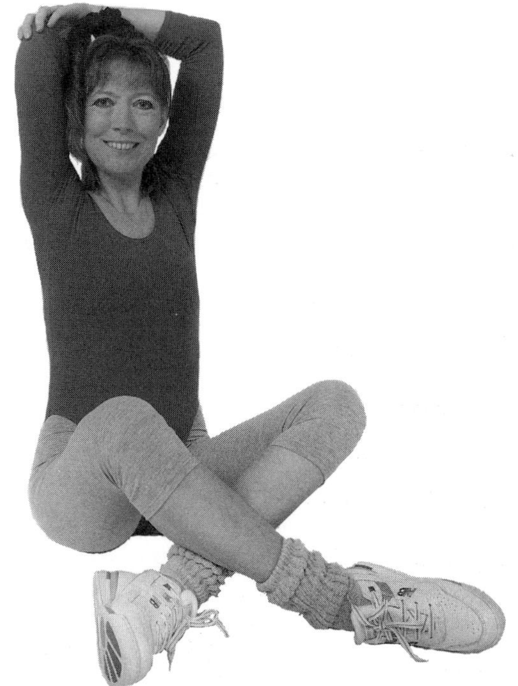

Cool-down Stretches (continued) ▶

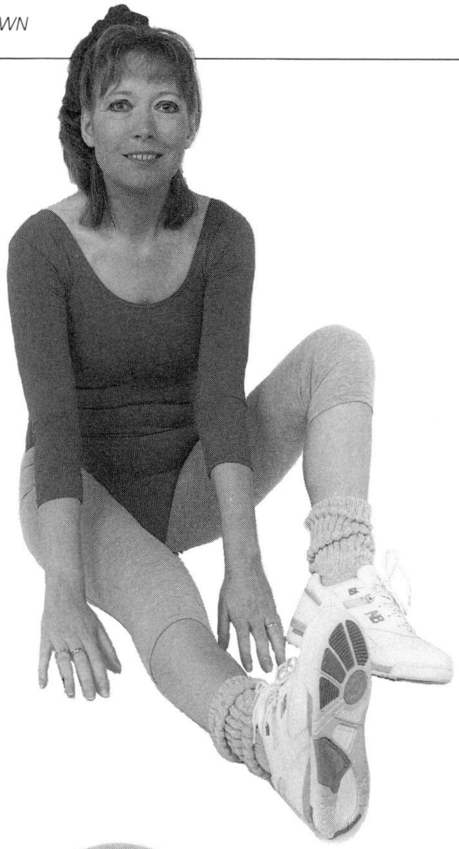

5. Sitting hamstring stretch

Sit on floor with left leg bent and left foot on floor in a comfortable position. Stretch right leg out in front of you.

Keeping back straight, lean forward over the right leg and place hands either side of leg.

Lean into the stretch until you feel the back of the upper thigh (hamstring) working.

Repeat the stretch to the other side. Over the weeks, aim to get your body lower down over the straight leg, again without arching back.

6. Hip and waist stretch

Lie on your back and bring your right leg over your body to lie on the floor on your left. Stretch arms out and bring head to right so that you feel a stretch in your right hip and bottom, and in your left waist.

Repeat to other side.

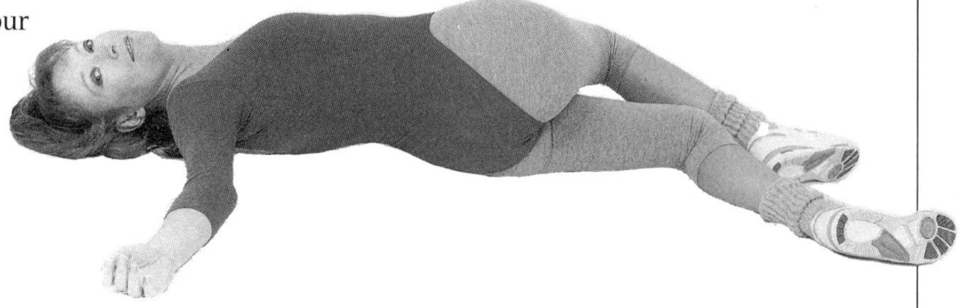

7. Long body stretch

Lie on back, stretching arms out above head. Breathe slowly and deeply as you elongate your whole body, stretching out waist area, rib cage and hips (wriggle legs down further if necessary as you stretch out).

Keep bottom quite taut and feet flexed once you are at full stretch.

Stay there as long as you like.

When you have finished the stretches, get up slowly and circle your arms around, stepping from side to side, for a few seconds.

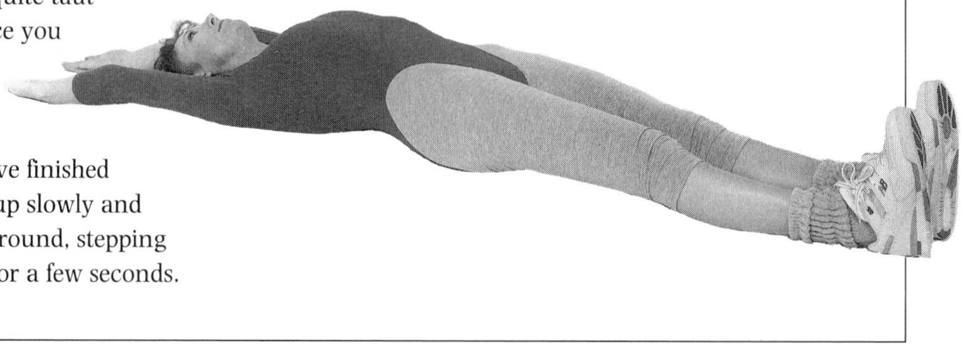

Supplement 1: Bust/chest, upper back and arms

1. Press-ups

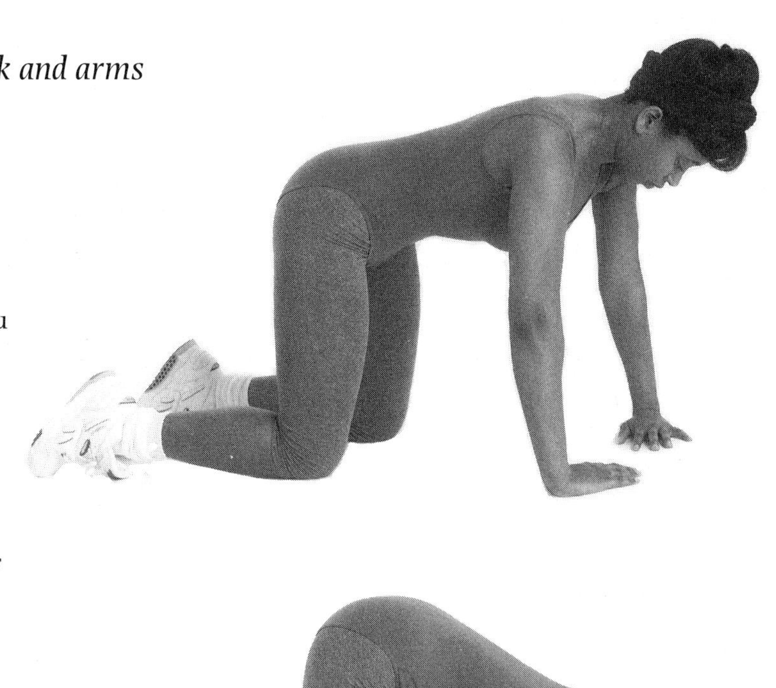

When you start press-ups, you'll probably be surprised how weak your arms are. Just do what you can, to start with.

Kneel on all fours as shown, with tummy tucked in and back not dipped in the centre. Have hands placed just out beyond shoulders to either side.

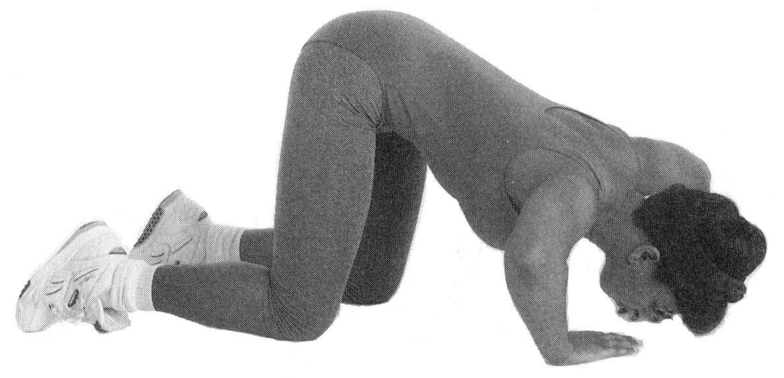

Now dip down towards the floor – touch it, if you can, with your forehead – and smoothly rise up again.

Do 8 press-ups, or as many as you can manage.

If doing further sets, rest between sets.

To make the press-ups harder, as you improve, take your knees further back and/or your arms wider apart. You can also dip with your head further forward.

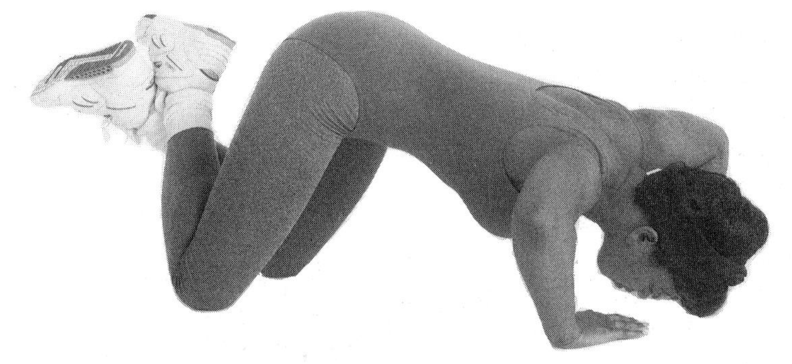

Supplement 1 (continued) ▶

2. Lying arm presses

Lie on your back on a mat with knees bent and lower back pressed firmly into the floor, arms out to sides.

Make fists and firmly bring your arms up so that they meet (from hand to elbow) above your chest. Hold for count of two, return and repeat 8 times for one set.

This exercise is much more effective if you wear wrist weights, or if you hold small hand weights.

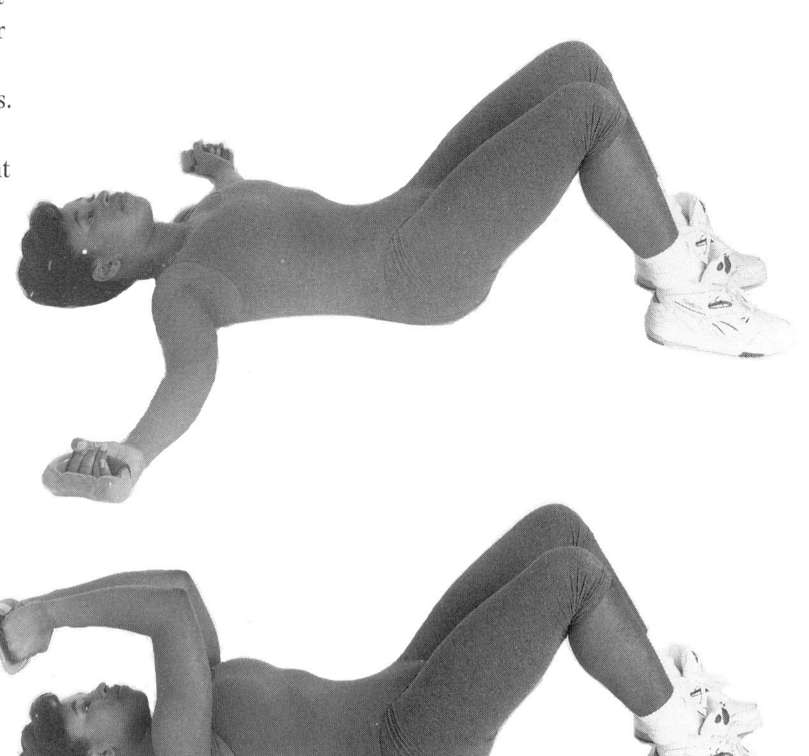

3. Upper back strengthener

Lie on your tummy on a mat with arms folded and hands under forehead. Breathing in, lift your shoulders, neck and head off the floor as far as you can. Count to one, and slowly relax to floor.

Repeat 8 times. You may find you can only come a tiny way off the floor to start with, but persist; you will soon improve.

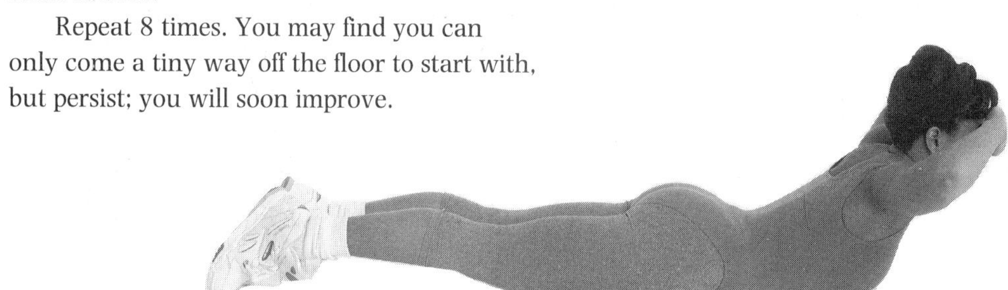

Supplement 1 (continued) ▶

4. Biceps curls

Stand with feet hip-width apart, knees slightly bent and tummy tucked in. Hold light weights in each hand, with palms facing outwards as shown. Keeping elbows tight in to hips, bring left weight up to shoulder.

Very *slowly* lower weight back down to start and repeat with other hand.

Repeat 8 times. This exercise can be done without weights, but it is not nearly so effective.

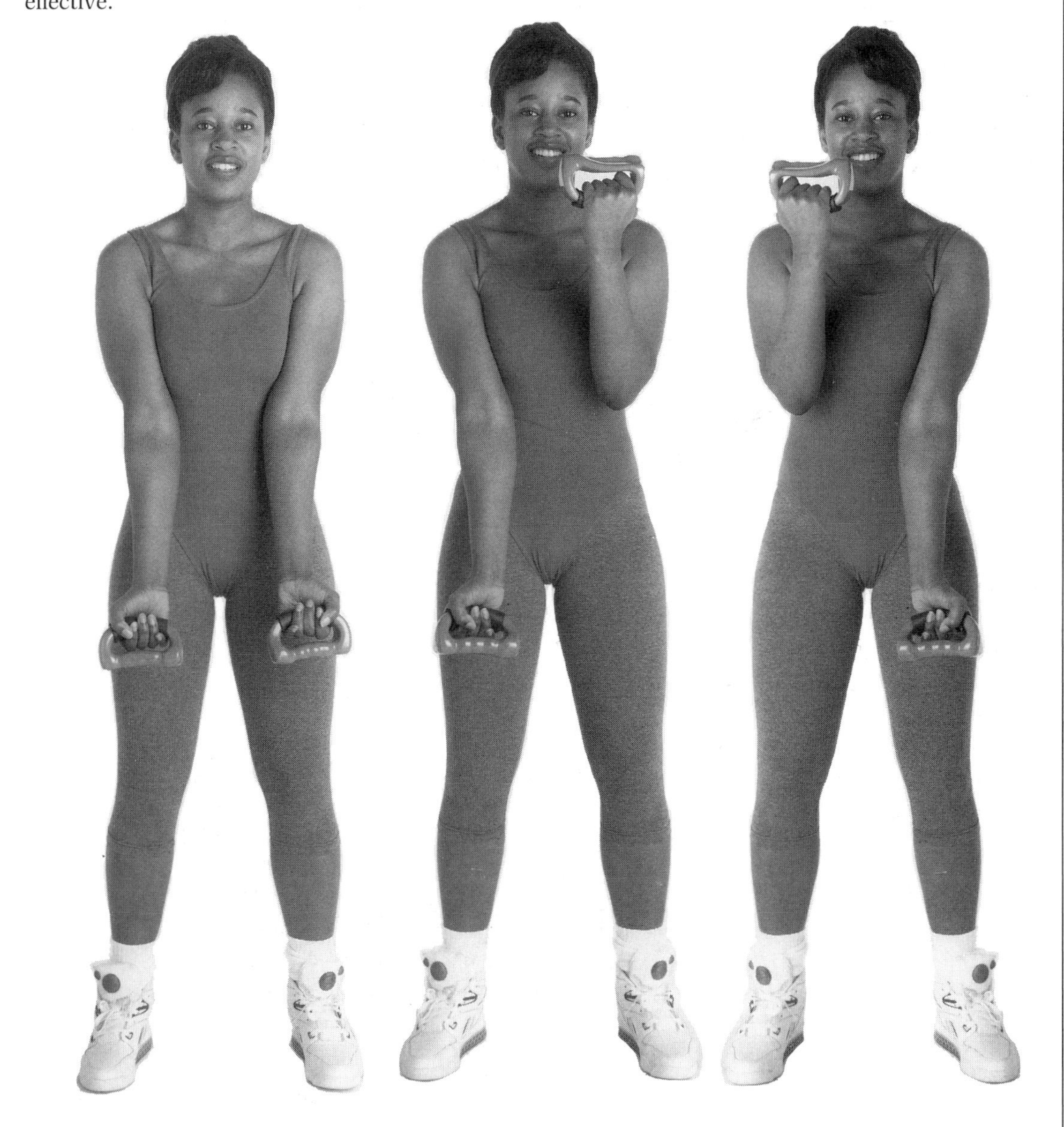

Supplement 2: Waist and stomach

1. Stomach crunches

Lie on your back with knees bent, stomach pressed flat to floor and hands placed at sides of head. Cross ankles and bring feet off floor.

Breathing out, lift head and shoulders off floor and at the same time bring knees in to meet head.

Inhale as you relax, and repeat 8 times.

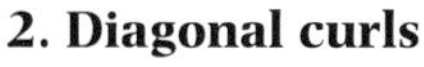

2. Diagonal curls

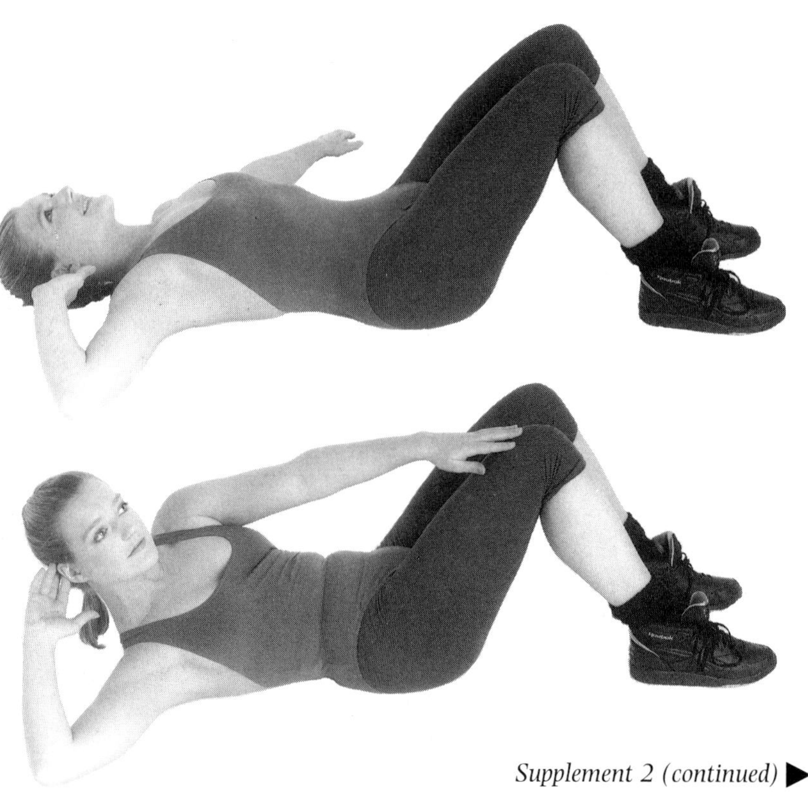

Lie on your back with knees bent and lower back flat on the floor. With right hand on right ear and right elbow on floor, bring head and left shoulder off floor, bring left arm over and touch outside of right knee.

Slowly return to start and repeat 8 times.

Repeat to other side.

Supplement 2 (continued) ▶

3. Curl ups II

Lie on back on floor with knees bent, lower back flat on floor and hands at sides of head. Breathing out, lift head and shoulders off floor and as you do so, bring right knee in, bringing head slightly to the right.

Slowly lower leg and head, and repeat, bringing left leg in this time and bringing head slightly to the left.

Do 8 repeats each side alternately.

When you are stronger you can do the movement a little more quickly by not returning each leg to the floor, and keeping the non-working leg raised.

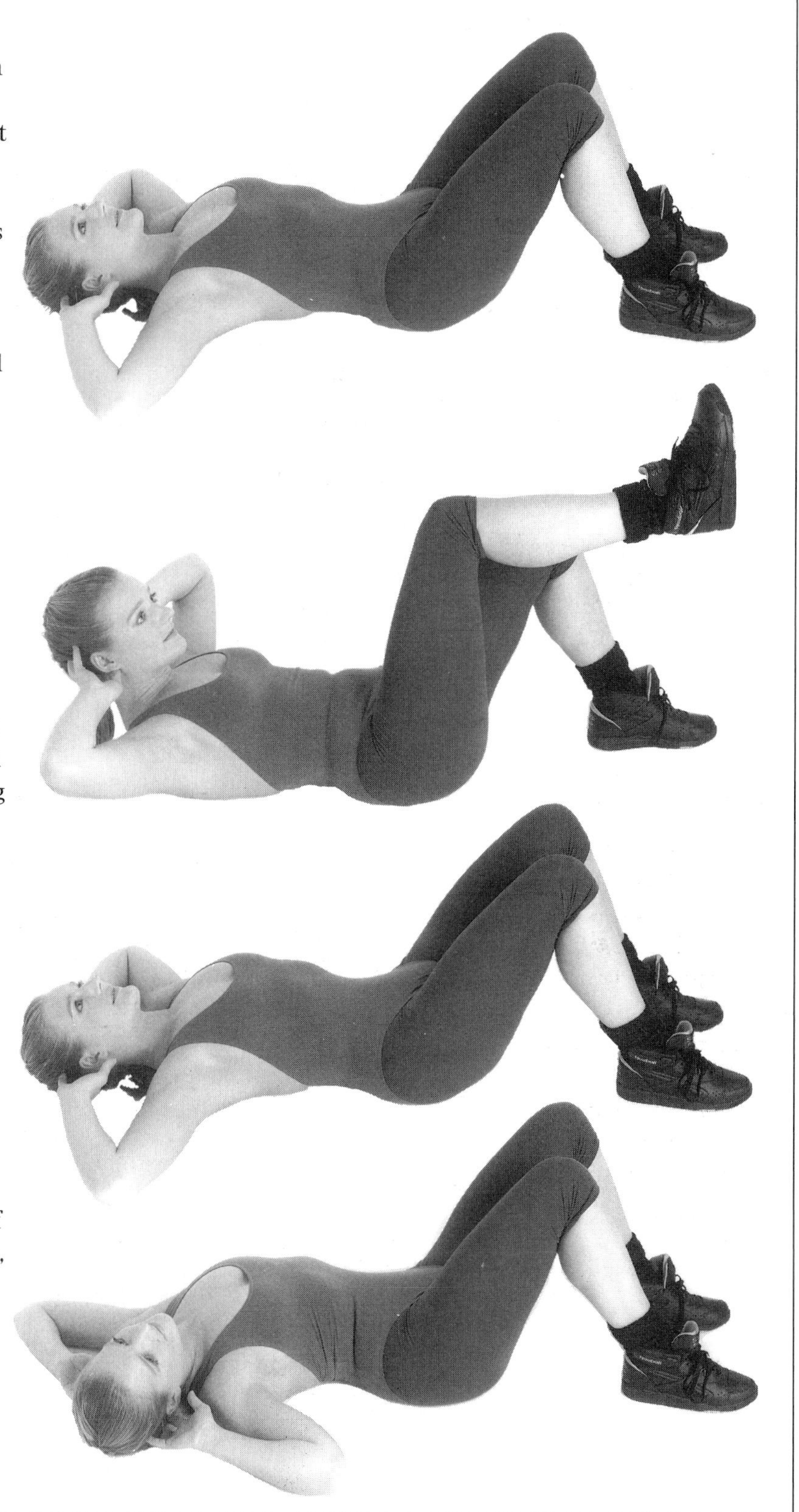

4. Lying side stretch

Lie on back, knees bent and hands at sides of head. Bring upper body slowly round to right, keeping it flat on the floor, until you feel a good stretch along the left waist.

Hold for the count of ten, move back to centre, and repeat to left side.

This is a stretch rather than a strengthening exercise, but it is excellent to define waist.

Supplement 3: Bottom and hips

1. Kneeling leg lifts

Kneel with upper body weight supported on forearms, and with tummy tucked in. Straighten right leg and bring it in line with back.

Keeping foot flexed, slowly move right leg up and down a few inches either way.

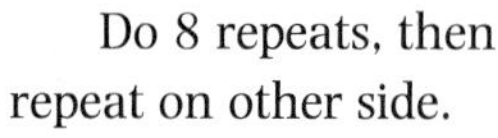

Do 8 repeats, then repeat on other side.

This exercise is also good for the lower back, and for firming the backs of the thighs.

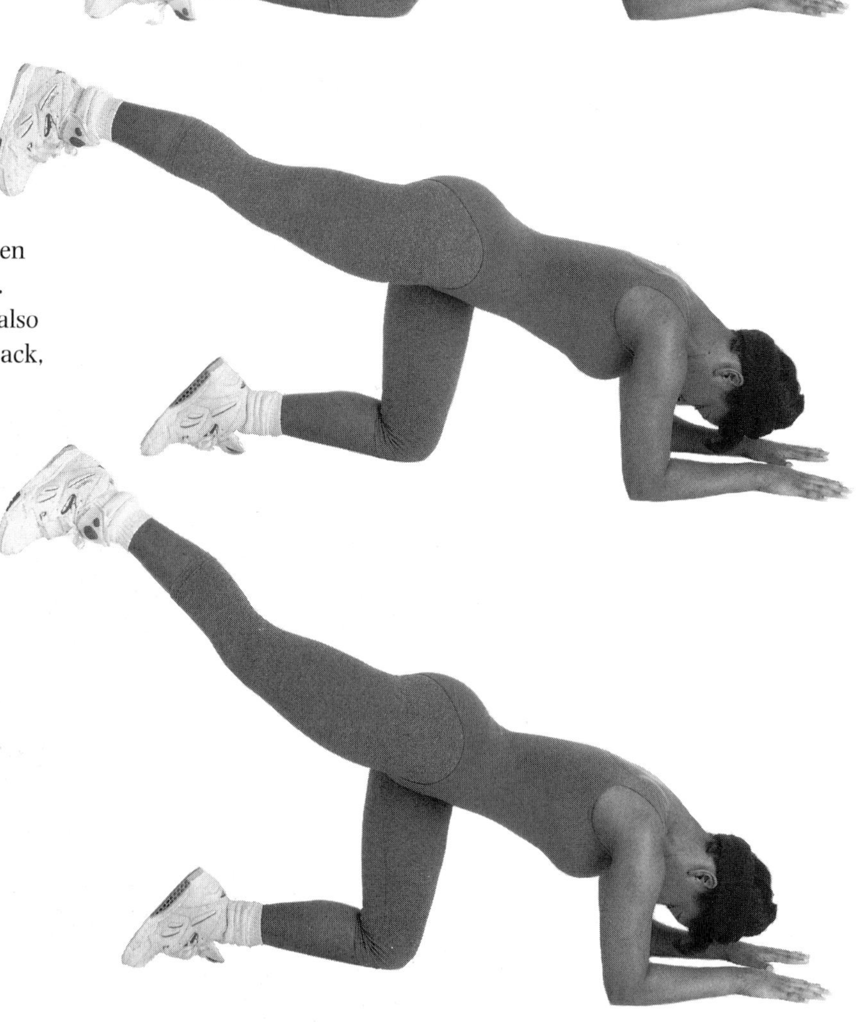

Supplement 3 (continued) ▶

2. Hip rotations

Lie on your left side with upper-body weight supported on left arm, right hand in front of body, left leg bent as shown.

Raise right leg, keeping knee slightly bent, to approximately 1 ft (30 cm) off floor, and slowly rotate it clockwise (to the back as far as it will go, feeling the hip and bottom of the right leg working).

Rotate the foot (keeping it flexed) forward and back 8 times, drop the leg, rest ten seconds then repeat another 8 times.

Turn over and work the left leg in the same way.

This exercise will also tone the thighs a little.

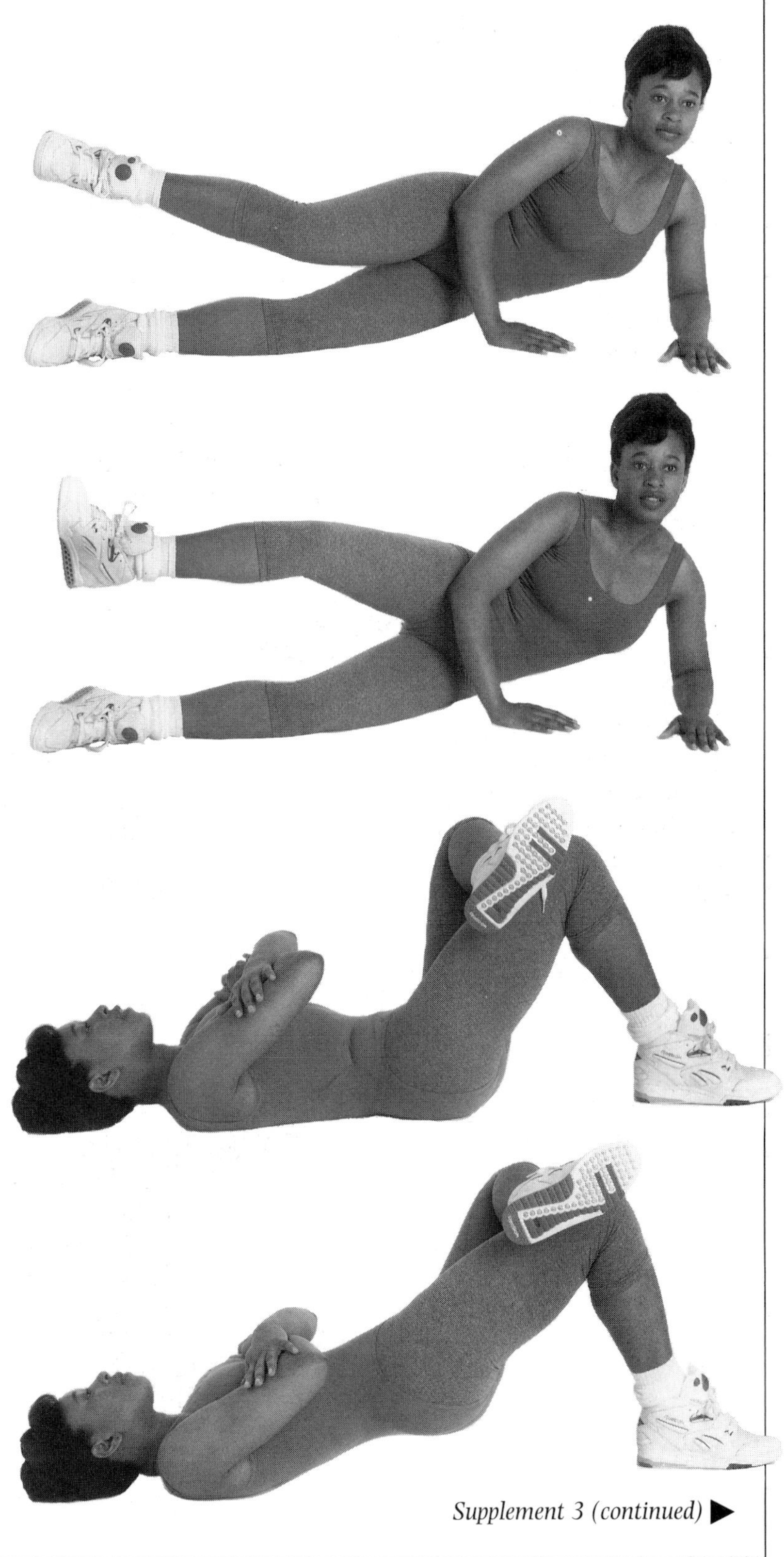

3. Crossed leg bottom squeezes

Lie on your back with knees bent, feet on floor, lower back pressed into floor, arms crossed over chest. Now bring left leg up and cross it over right leg, as shown, so that left foot hangs loose.

Using bottom strength, squeeze and lift lower body off floor.

Slowly return to start and repeat 8 times; repeat to other side.

The added weight of your crossed leg makes this exercise very effective.

Supplement 3 (continued) ▶

4. Side leg raises

Kneel on all fours with legs hip-width apart, tummy tucked in. Now, very slowly, keeping knee bent, bring right leg up to the side until knee is approximately one foot (30 cm) off floor (or lower).

Slowly lower and repeat 8 times.

Repeat with left leg.

Don't try to go too far on this movement; don't do it quickly.

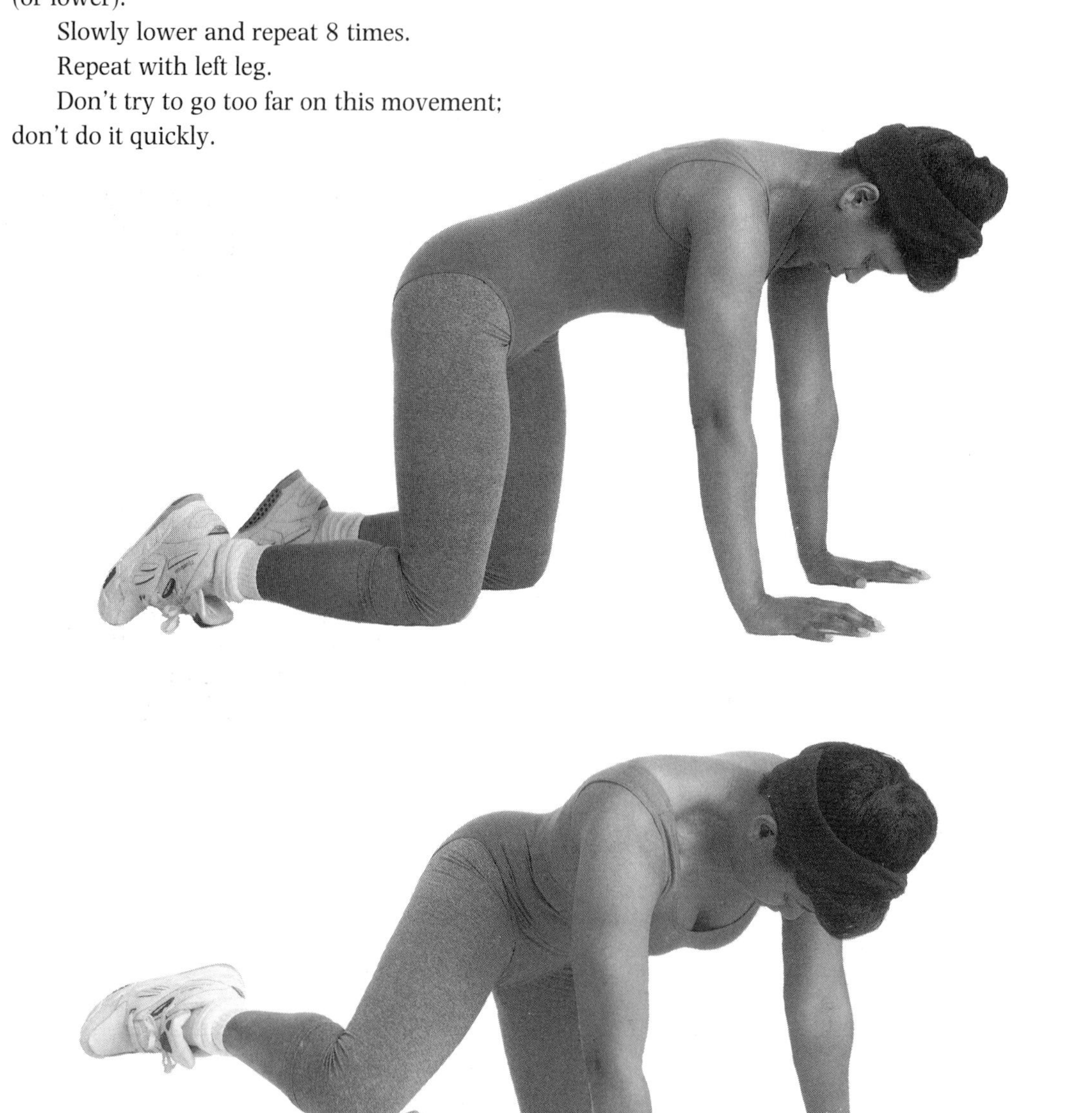

Supplement 4: Thighs and calves

1. Inner thigh lift

Lie on right side as shown, with left foot on floor in front of right leg.

Keeping hips upright and still, and keeping foot flexed, lift right leg as high as it will go, then slowly return to floor.

Repeat 8 times.

Repeat on other side.

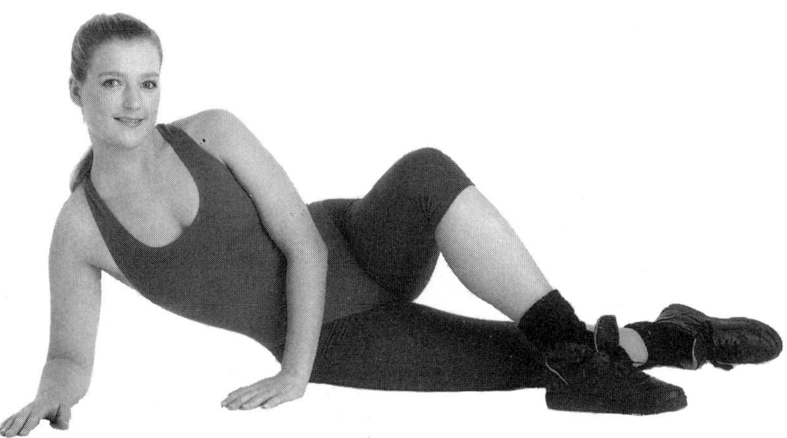

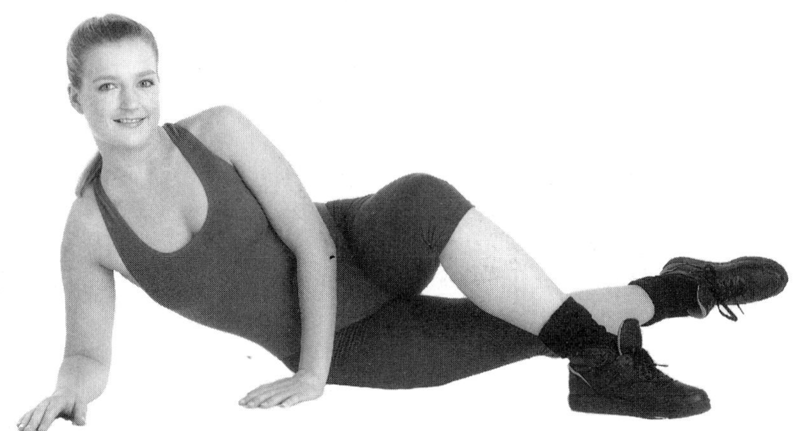

When your inner thigh is stronger, you can make this exercise harder by placing the calf of your left leg on top of your right leg to add resistance.

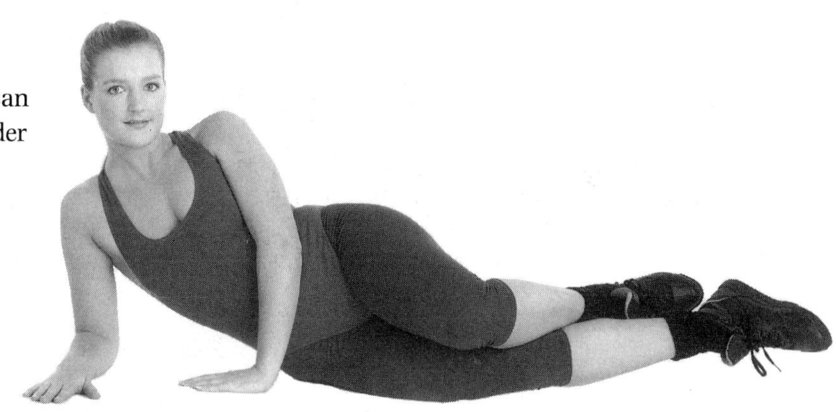

Supplement 4 (continued) ▶

2. Hamstring strengthener

Kneel as shown, keeping tummy tucked in.

Raise right leg until it is horizontal to floor. Now, slowly bend right knee and, keeping thigh still, bring lower leg up and as far in towards your bottom as you can.

Hold for the count of one. Slowly return to start and repeat 8 times.

Repeat to other side.

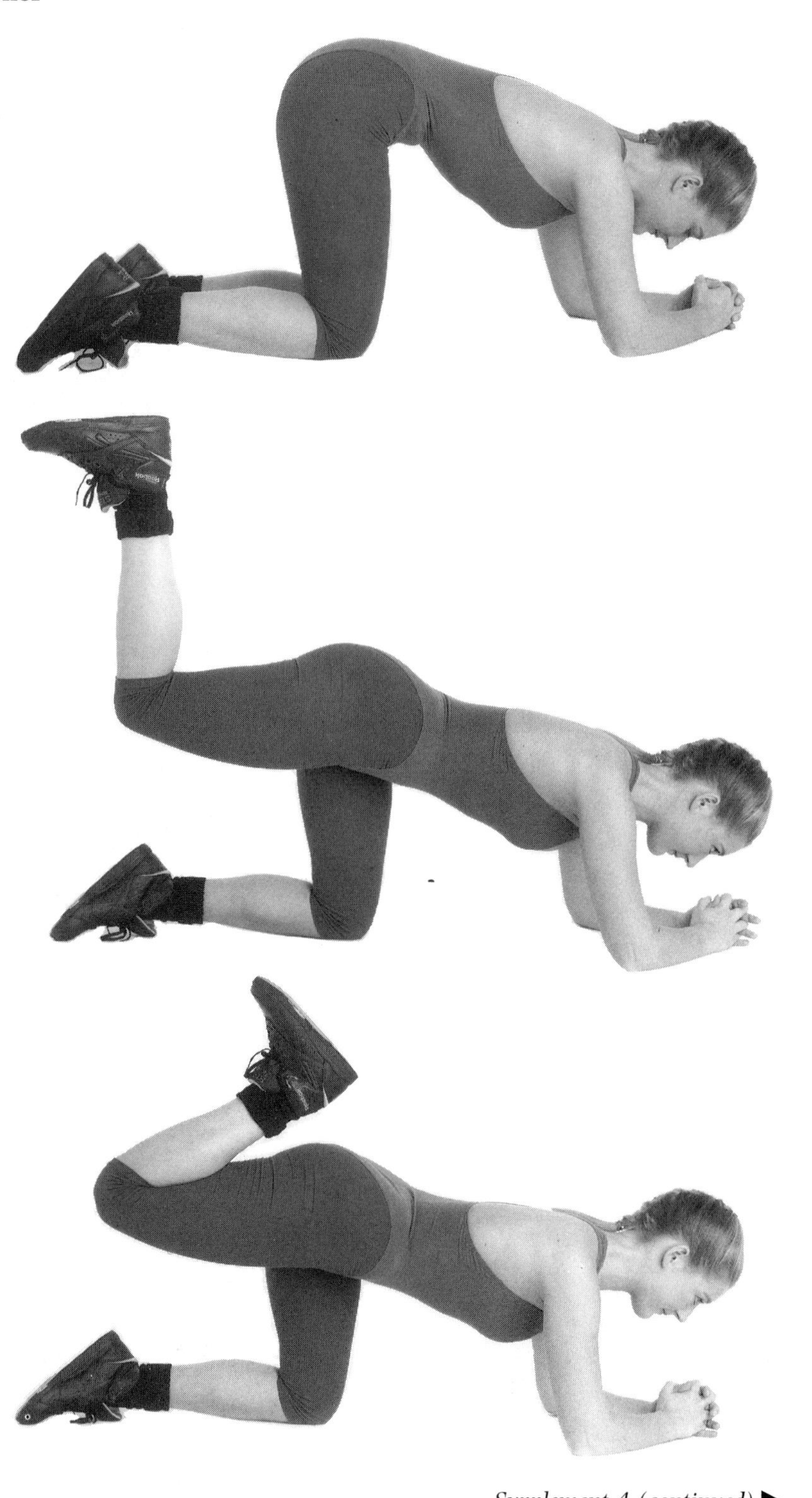

Supplement 4 (continued) ▶

3. Lying side leg raises

Lie on left side with body weight supported as shown and left leg bent.

Keeping hips square to the front, raise right leg until it is approximately 18 ins (45 cm) off the floor.

Keeping right foot flexed and toe facing forwards, lift right foot up approximately 9 ins (22.5 cm), hold for the count of one, then slowly lower 9 ins (22.5 cm).

Repeat 8 times without lowering right leg back down to floor, and keeping leg straight.

Turn over and repeat other side.

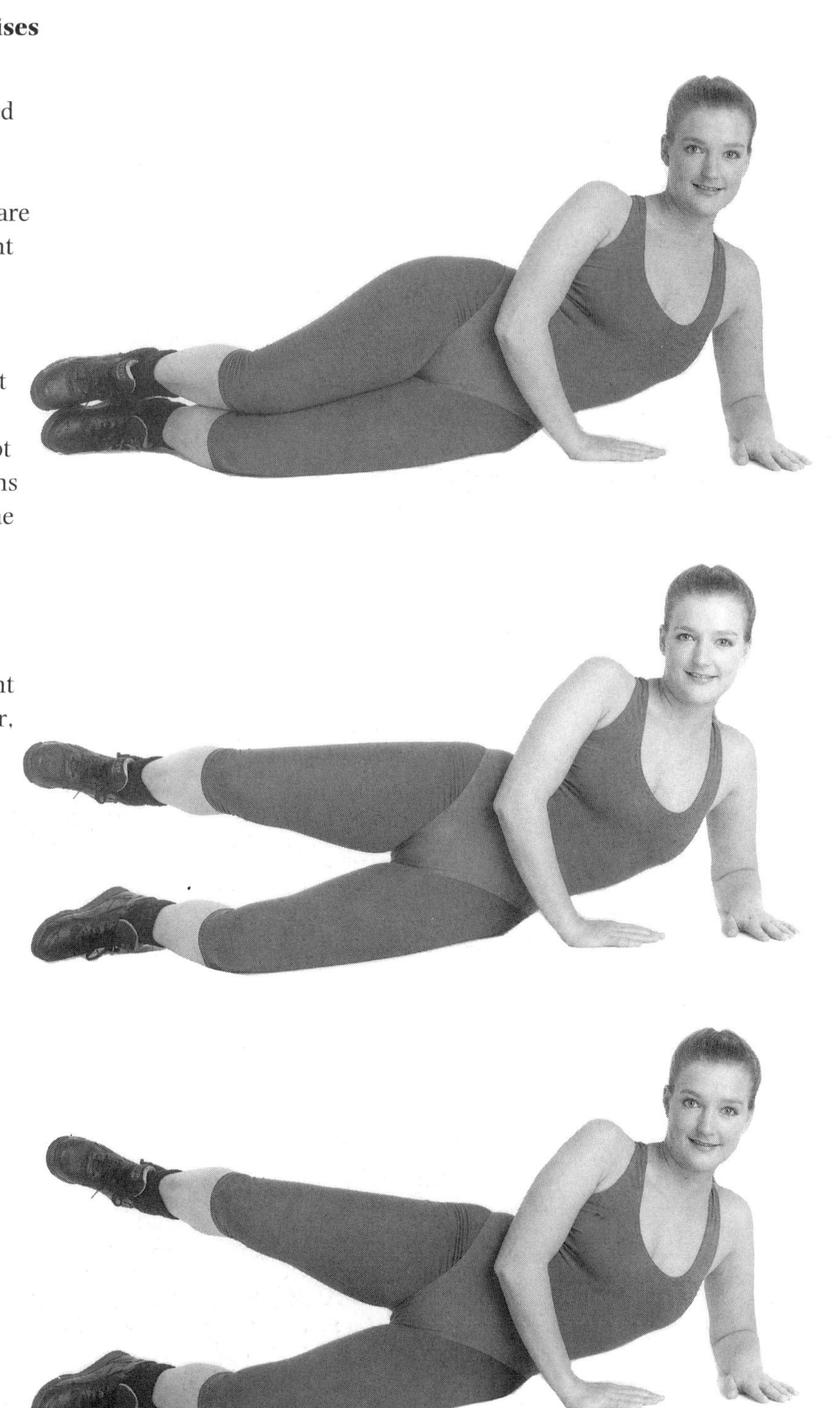

Supplement 4 (continued) ▶

4. Calf raises with half-squats

Stand with feet approximately 2 ft (60 cm) apart, knees bent, tummy tucked in, toes in line with knees, hands lightly resting on hips.

Now bend into a half-squat as shown, keeping back straight and shoulders in line with knees and ankles, maintaining good balance. While in the squat, raise left heel and then right heel as shown, come up out of the squat on toes and slowly lower heels to floor.

Repeat sequence 8 times. If you have trouble coming up on to your toes while in the squat, you could hold the edge of a chairback to help.

Or do 8 squats, then eight calf raises separately to begin with.

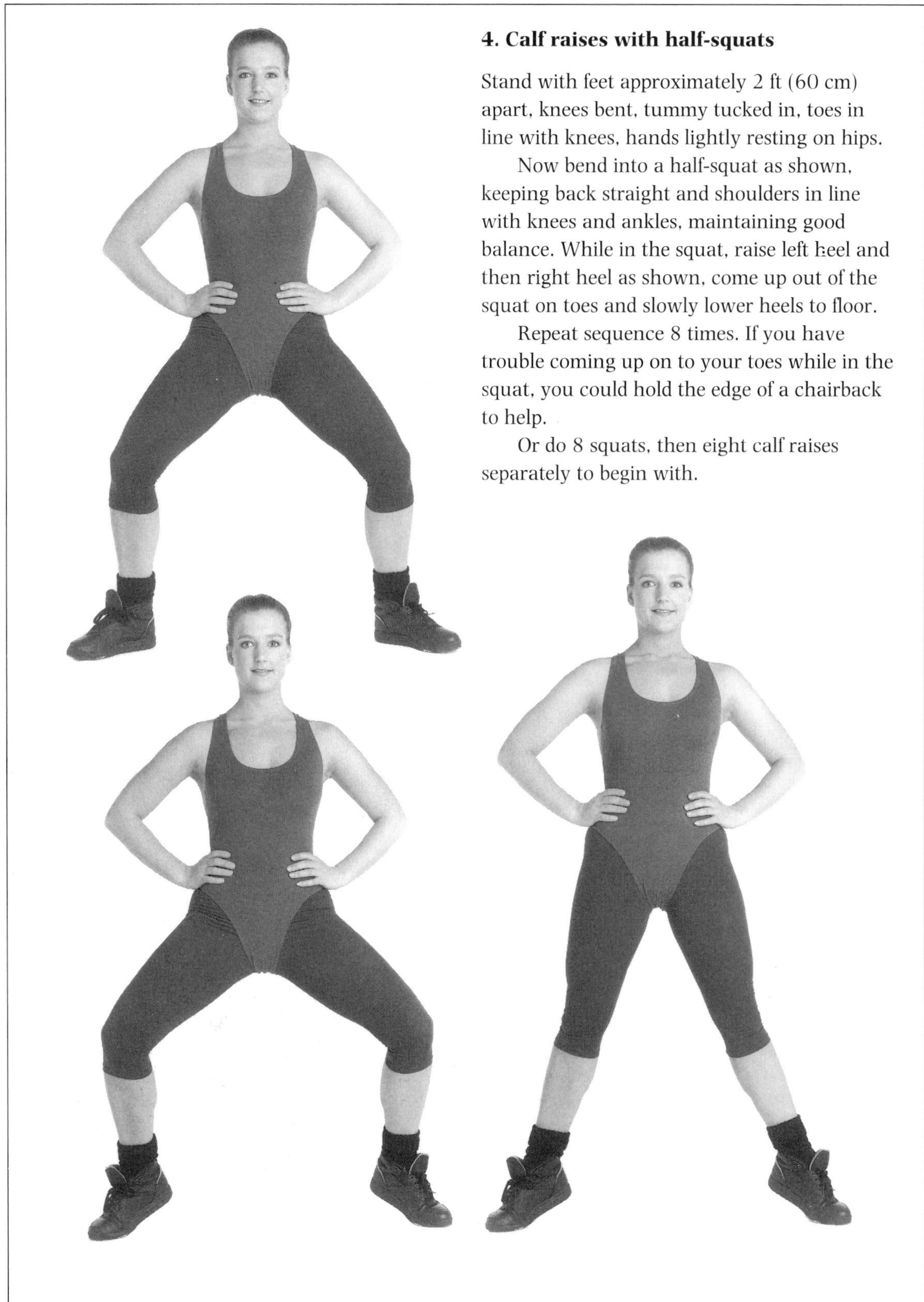

Supplement 5: Flexibility

1. Hip flexor, bottom and lower back stretch

Lie on back with lower back pressed into floor, bring right leg in to chest and clasp with both hands around front calf as shown.

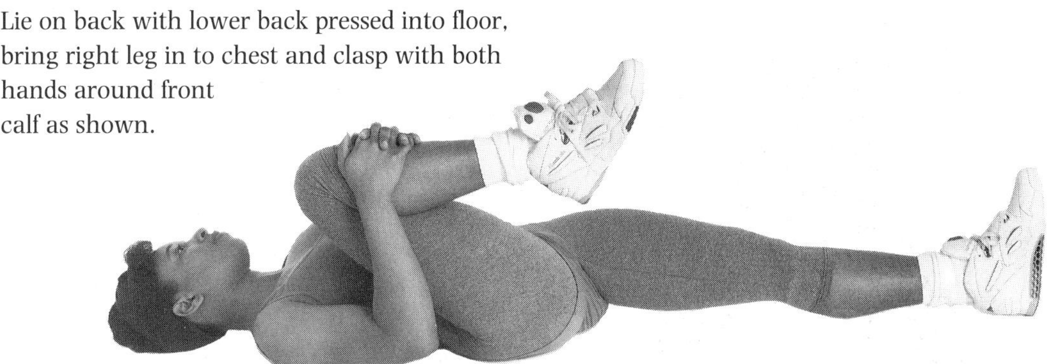

Slowly pull the bent leg towards your chest, all the while attempting to keep your left leg down on the floor. The harder you find this stretch, the more you need to stretch this area. It is best to keep the straight leg on the floor and gradually over the weeks bring your bent leg nearer the chest than vice versa.

Hold the stretch as far as it will go for 10 seconds, building up to 30 seconds.

2. Hamstring stretch

Lie on back as in Exercise 1 but this time with both knees bent. Bring right leg in and clasp it around the back of the thigh.

Gently pull back to feel the hamstring stretch. Keep knee bent. Hold for 10 seconds, building up to 30 seconds.

Over the weeks you may find you can straighten out the leg.

Repeat to other side.

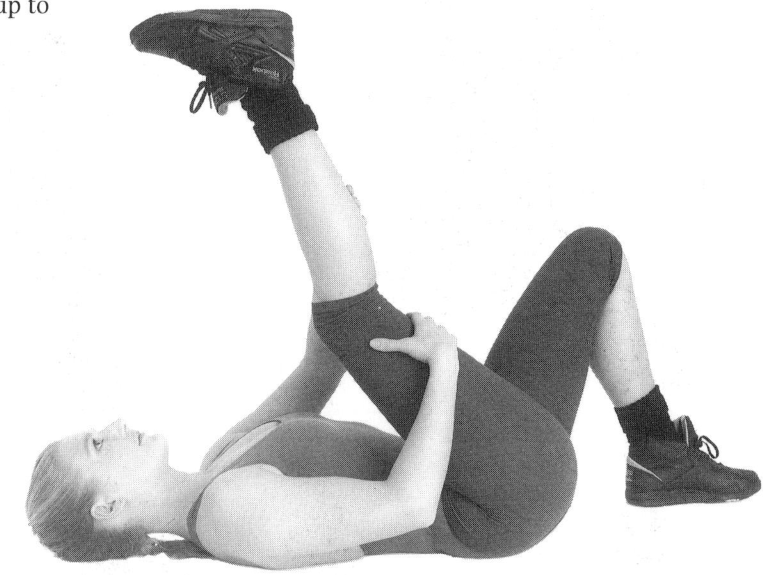

Supplement 5 (continued) ▶

3. Groin and inner thigh stretch

Sit on mat with back straight and legs bent so that feet have soles together and are about 1 ft (30 cm) in front of your groin.

Clasp ankles with hands, as shown, and using your elbows, press gently down on inside of knees to lower knees towards floor.

Hold at the maximum stretch for 10 seconds, building up to 30 seconds.

As your inner thighs and groin loosen up, you will be able to bring your feet closer in towards your groin and your knees will come nearer to the floor.

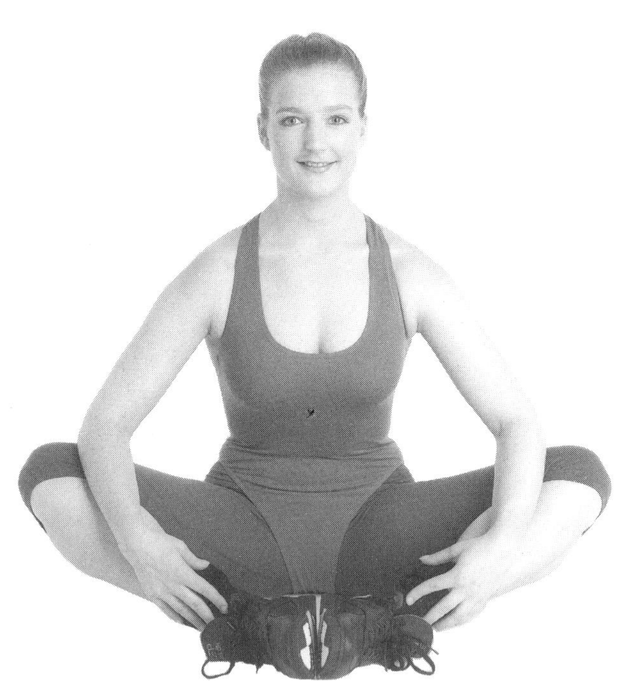

4. Back twist

This stretch will help to mobilise a tight back. Sit on mat with right leg bent as shown, and left leg crossed over it so that left foot is on floor beyond
right knee.

Placing left hand on floor behind left hip, move upper body round to look over towards the left as far back as you can.

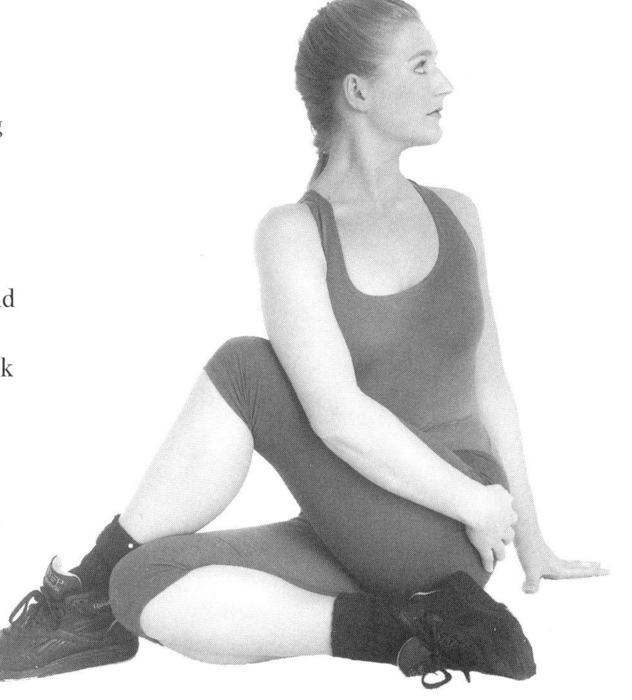

Supplement 5 (continued) ▶

5. Chest stretch

Lie on back on mat with knees bent. Bring arms out to the sides up to head level, keeping elbows bent and palms up.

Keep lower back firm into floor and feel a stretch across your chest.

Hold for 10 seconds, building up to 30 seconds.

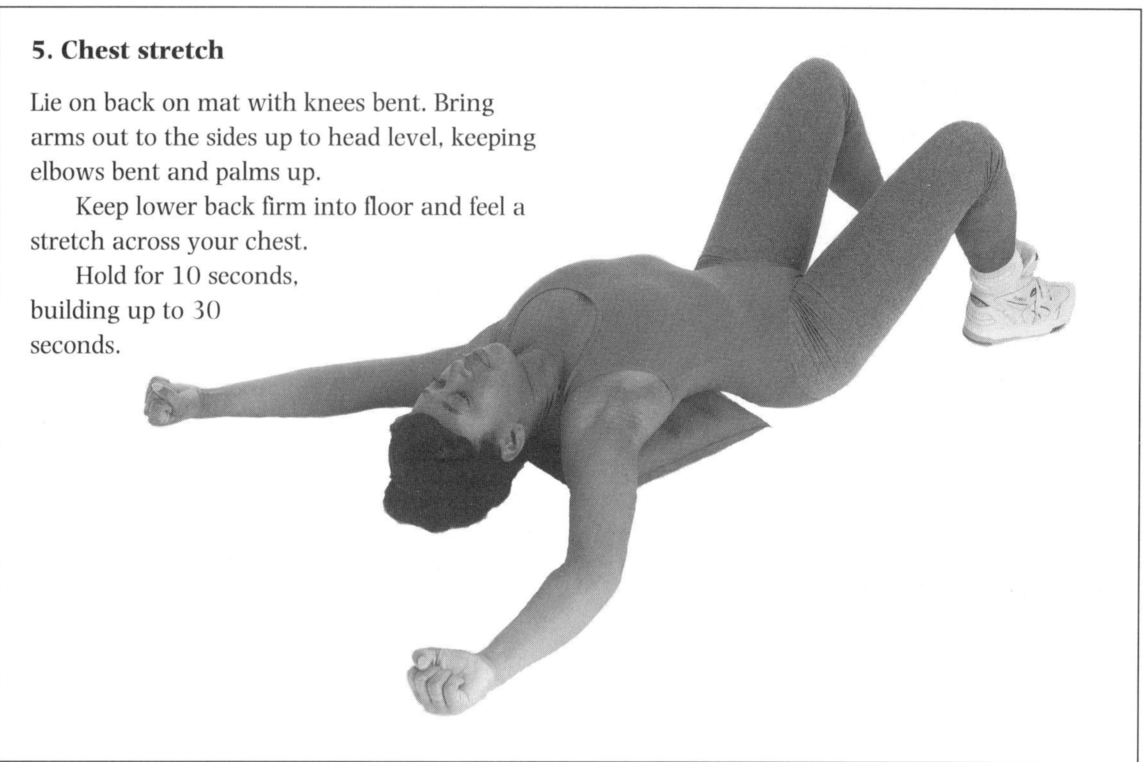

STAYING SLIM 10

You've reached the weight and shape you want to be. I hope you're feeling proud of yourself. Now, you need to learn how to stabilise your weight at its new level. There is no physical reason why you ever have to put that fat back on again unless, that is, you return to the eating habits and sedentary lifestyle that made you overweight to begin with.

Don't worry, you won't find it hard to keep in shape now... and always. With the help of the 'transition phase', the practical and psychological tips in this chapter, and the exclusive food charts that tell you all you need to know about any food at a glance, you will find that staying slim is no problem at all.

THE TRANSITION PHASE

Just as the Speed Slimming Diet System took you *down* a sliding scale of calories as you lost weight, so the Transition Phase slides you back up. You gradually eat more, over a period of twelve days, after which time you are ready to start taking complete control of your own diet.

This transition phase has two main benefits:

- It helps to prevent that 'Yippee, I'm off the diet' madness that overcomes so many people, prompting them to rush round and eat everything in sight without thought.
- It helps to avoid the sudden glycogen gain. This is the three to four pound (1.4–1.8 kg) weight gain that happens to anyone who suddenly eats a lot more than usual. It isn't fat returning but a mixture of glucose and water, the same thing that you lost quickly in the first week of your diet (see page 17).

Although the return of glycogen is natural and unavoidable – and, most importantly, it isn't fat – it can be very discouraging to witness a sudden weight gain over a period of a day or two. The transition phase gives you an extra twelve days of 'semi-diet', so that while the glycogen gradually returns, you are still losing a little body fat. Therefore, at the end of the twelve days, the fat loss/glycogen gain should even out, and you should end up weighing the same as you did at the start of the twelve-day period.

How it works

The transition phase is simplicity itself. You will have finished your diet on Diet 5. For the next twelve days, you:

- Spend the first three days on Diet 4;
- Spend the next three days on Diet 3;
- Spend the next three days on Diet 2; and
- Spend the final three days on Diet 1.

By the time you reach Day 12, you will be eating 1500 calories a day. During the twelve days, you can choose menus from any three days in the plan you're working from. Or, you can follow the flexi diet, and mix and match menus.

PLANNING YOUR OWN DIET

At the end of the transition phase, you are ready to begin taking complete control of what and how much you eat.

Female readers, your weight-maintenance calorie level will be approximately 2000 a day (perhaps more), assuming that you follow the exercise and lifestyle maintenance tips below. Male readers can expect a maintenance level of 2500 calories. The good news is, however, that you *don't* have to count every calorie for the rest of your life in order to stay slim.

All you need to do is remember this tip.

The more *fat* you reduce in your diet, and the more *complex carbohydrates* you eat, the more likely you are to stay slim for life.

This will work for you for four reasons:

- As you read in Chapter 1, a high-carbohydrate intake actually helps your metabolic rate to stay high. You burn up more calories if you eat carbohydrate than you do if you eat fat.
- If you eat plenty of complex carbohydrates, fruit and vegetables, you won't feel as hungry.
- If you restrict fats, you will automatically be restricting calories, because at nine calories per gram (that's about one-fifth of a level teaspoon), fat contains more than double the calories of either protein or carbohydrate.
- If you eat plenty of complex carbohydrates, you will feel full up long before you get to the stage of eating enough calories to make you fat.

In other words, both over-eating and being overweight, on a diet that contains the right proportions of fat, carbohydrate and protein, is almost impossible. So, if you continue to fill up your plate with high-carbohydrate, starchy foods (such as potatoes, rice, pasta and bread), plus vegetables and fruit, you will *never* have a problem with hunger and you *never* need to put on weight again.

Look at it this way. You could have a 1 oz (25 g) pat of butter for 200 calories. Or, you could have a 6 oz (175 g) baked potato, topped with 2 oz (50 g) baked beans for 200 calories. Need I say more?

So how much carbohydrate is enough, and how much fat is too much?

In Britain we currently eat up to forty per cent of our diet in the form of fat, but the World Health Organisation (WHO) suggests that for good health (and weight restriction) we should limit our fat intake to a maximum of thirty per cent of our total energy (calorie) intake.

For lifelong slimness, an even better figure to aim for is between twenty and twenty-five per cent. On a maintenance diet of, say, 2000 calories, that still represents between 400 and 500 daily calories of fats (and oils). Enough to give a great deal of leeway to any diet.

The WHO suggests a daily protein intake of between ten and fifteen per cent of our total energy (calorie) intake. And that leaves between sixty and seventy per cent of our calories to be eaten in the form of carbohydrates.

Complex, starchy carbohydrates, plus fresh fruit and vegetables, should form the bulk of this carbohydrate intake. Common sugar (table sugar, honey, syrup, treacle, glucose and all those sugars refined and added to biscuits, cakes, puddings, etc.) is also a carbohydrate, as we discussed in Chapter 1. However, it is linked more than any other food with dental caries; it doesn't have the long-term filling power of complex carbohydrates, it contains absolutely no nutrients and is often combined with lots of fat in manufactured goods.

Currently, virtually *half* of our carbohydrate intake is in the form of common sugars. The WHO recommends that we have no more than ten per cent of our daily calories in the form of common sugars; for weight maintenance, five to ten per cent is a good target to aim for.

So let's now compare the proportions of what your old-style diet (the one that made you fat) looks like, with your new-style diet, the one that will keep you slim.

	OLD DIET (%)	NEW DIET (%)
fat	40	20–25
protein	15	10–15
carbohydrate	45 total *	60–70 †

* (22.5% complex carbohydrates, vegetables and fruit; 22.5% simple sugars).

† (maximum 10% of total energy should be from common sugars).

Putting theory into practice

You've been practising the carbo/fat balancing trick all the time you've been losing weight on the Complete Speed Slimming System. With a little more practice you will easily do the same on your maintenance diet. In fact, the proportions on the slimming diet plans were a little tougher than are necessary now. Fat content on the diets works out at a little *less* than twenty per cent fat on average, and simple carbohydrates (sugars) were never more than 7.5 % per unit.

You have enjoyed meals based on these principles on the Complete Speed Slimming System, and you'll continue to do so. There is no reason at all why you can't enjoy a lifetime of tasty, tempting low-fat high-carbohydrate meals.

As a back-up system, I have devised the new, unique food charts at the end of this chapter. I have worked out for you the percentages of fat calories and carbohydrate calories in almost all of our everyday foods, so it is very easy to see at a glance how well any particular food measures up to the carbo/fat balance.

The following tips will help you keep off that weight.

- Once you begin to plan your full maintenance diet, the simplest way to start is to choose meals and extras similar to the meals in Diet 1. Increase portion sizes by around twenty-five per cent, particularly the complex carbohydrate foods: bread, potatoes, pasta, rice and pulses. This is a very easy way to take your daily calories up to a maintenance level, while keeping fat low.
- Once you are used to that, you could begin to add your own favourite foods to your menu. First, look them up in the food charts (pages 126 –143) and then decide how they should be added. Are they high in fat? Restrict them to small portions, or an occasional treat.
- Plan every meal – breakfast, lunch and evening – around a high-complex-carbohydrate food. For example, decide whether the basis of your meal will be a baked potato, rice, pasta, pulses, or bread. To that, add a little low-fat high-protein food, if necessary (e.g. white fish, poultry, low-fat yoghurt, etc.). Many carbohydrate foods also contain plenty of protein (all pulses do, for instance).

You should get into the habit of using the low-fat vegetable protein foods (such as baked beans or lentil soup) rather than thinking you've got to have the higher-fat protein sources, such as red meat or hard cheese.

- Add to your plate plenty of fresh vegetables or salad, and follow with fresh fruit.
- If you enjoy making recipe dishes rather than eating 'plain' food, try to make more use of ingredients such as herbs, spices, and the oriental seasonings like sweet and sour sauces, rather than relying on oil and butter in large quantities. Follow the methods and cooking ideas in the recipes in the Complete Speed Slimming System – you'll find plenty of ideas on how to keep the taste while keeping fat content low.

Between meals, snack, on high-carbohydrate items such as bananas, bread and dried fruits.

If the majority of your daily calorie intake is based on the above tips, then you can safely add some 'extras'. Remember, something that you eat only occasionally – say, once every week or two – is unlikely to make any real difference to your weight. So if there is a really high fat food that you simply *must* have now and then – have it. A chocolate bar once a week or so isn't going to make you fat. But if you want chocolate every day- either have just a couple of squares of a bar, or a 'funsize' bar, or how about getting that chocolatey taste another, lower-fat way – say a low-fat instant chocolate drink.

- Don't forget that fat isn't just things like butter, margarine and cooking oil. Fat is a hidden ingredient in many, many foods, particularly dairy produce, meats, manufactured sweet and savoury foods, pastries, nuts and crisps. Your total fat intake will consist of everything you eat that has fat in it. For your health, it is better to eat the vegetable oils rather than saturated (dairy and animal) fats but as far as your waistline goes, both types contain similar calories. (Butter has a little less calories per ounce and less fat than oil because it has a water content).

People sometimes complain that they do eat a diet high in complex carbohydrates, but they still put on weight. I analyse what they are eating, and it usually turns out that they are adding lots of fat to their carbohydrate meals, without realising it. For instance, adding a rich, cream sauce to their pasta, or loads of full-fat Cheddar cheese to their baked potato.

So, I do urge you to *check the food charts* (see pages 126–143) before starting to plan your own diet. See just what *is* in your own favourite items, and it will probably give you a good clue as to why you had a weight problem in the first place.

To give you even more help, here are three 'favourite food' lists. List 1 itemises foods you can eat without thinking about them on your diet. List 2 is foods you should treat with a little caution (they have a little more fat and/or a little fewer carbohydrates). List 3 is the 'go carefully' list.

List 1
(Eat as much as you like.)

All fresh fruit
All fresh vegetables
Potatoes
Wholegrain breads
Other breads (but try to eat wholegrain)
Pasta (try to eat wholewheat)
Rice (try to eat brown)
All pulses (including beans, lentils, chick peas etc.)
Bulgar (cracked wheat)
Wholewheat breakfast cereals without added sugar
Low-fat crispbreads and rice cakes
Dried fruits

List 2
(Exercise a little caution. Don't eat too many of these at the expense of the high-carbohydrate low-fat items in List 1.)

Yoghurt
White fish
Prawns
Crab
Chicken
Game
Liver
Cottage cheese
Skimmed milk soft cheese
Vegetable burgers or bangers
Low-fat fromage frais
Skimmed milk
Eggs
Lean red meat
Muesli

Still List 2, but use a little more caution as the fat content is getting higher.

Fresh nuts and seeds
Whole milk yoghurt
Oily fish, fresh or canned
Avocado
Most tinned soups
Vegetable pâtés

List 3
(Go carefully)

Butter and all spreading fats
All salad and cooking oils
Salad dressing
Mayonnaise
All fatty cuts of meat, including sausages, shoulder of lamb, bacon and duck
Cream
High or medium-fat cheeses
Chips
Crisps and salted nuts
Pastry
Biscuits and cakes
Chocolates and sweets
Puddings
Deep fried foods

EXERCISE AND LIFESTYLE

To maintain your metabolism at a good, consistent, raised level, it is important that you continue to do some regular exercise. Exercise is also important to keep the shape that you've finally attained. Muscles soon disappear if you don't use them.

The exercise maintenance programme is simple.

Fat Burning Programme

Do your fat burning programme *three* times a week (more if you want to). This should be at the highest level you have attained during the fat burning programme in Chapter 3. (If that level was less than Standard 9, you could, of course, continue to improve until you do reach Standard 9.)

Body Shaping Programme

Do the *basic* routine twice a week (more if you want to). This is the minimum necessary to keep the shape you want. When you've finished slimming, if you still feel there is room for more shape improvement, you can, of course, continue doing the basic routine up to six times a week until you are happy with your shape.

If you were doing any supplement(s), continue them once a week, following a basic routine.

Other Activity

Consider giving more of your time to energetic activities; for instance, outdoor pursuits such as hiking or orienteering, canoeing or rock climbing! Now you're fit and slim, make the most of the new you to learn and enjoy new pursuits.

The same goes for sports; how about joining a local team, such as netball or hockey or football?

Always think 'active', that way you will continue to burn up plenty of calories. A basic sound fitness routine will also keep your body in good health and help prevent too many common ailments (e.g., osteoporosis, arthritis, cardio-vascular disease) that beset us in later years.

Lastly, never forget all the lifestyle tips for keeping up your metabolism. Get plenty of fresh air, breathe deeply. Enjoy life. Most of all, enjoy your food. Weigh yourself only once a week.

MIND OVER MATTER

THE PSYCHOLOGY OF WEIGHT MAINTENANCE

Planning out your diet and knowing what to eat is a very large part of successful weight maintenance, but it's by no means all of it. Your personality, feelings, moods, attitudes, habits and life events are all things that affect what you eat, and they can very quickly affect your weight.

So this section is to help you make sensible choices, even when you're sure you can't.

How much do you want to stay slim?

One of the best ways to help yourself stay slim for life is to know *why* you want to be slim. And the best way to find that out is to spend some quiet time with a pen and paper, writing down every single reason you can think of.

I've started you off with some ideas below. *You* fill in the rest of the list with your own. If you run out of room, list some more on plain paper. If the going ever gets tough, read this list and see just what you stand to lose.

I want to stay slim because:

- I have much more self-confidence in meeting people now that I'm slim.
- I feel fitter and am more energetic, now I am slim.
- I have so much more choice of clothes when I go shopping.
- ....
- ....
- ....

Hunger, or 'taste temptation'?

If you are hungry, you should always eat some good-quality fuel: never deny yourself. Occasionally, everyone eats something they fancy, not because they are hungry but just because that food looks – or smells – nice. One of the big differences between overweight and slim people is that fatties indulge *more* often in food *when they are not hungry*. If you learn to listen to your body, you will soon tell the difference.

You are likely to have one particular 'taste temptation'. It could be chocolate or biscuits, or cheese or salted nuts.

Think about this whole question of hunger, and fill in the blanks below.

These are the occasions I most often eat when I am not hungry:

....

....

....

....

These are the foods most likely to make me eat when I am not hungry:

....

....

....

....

Now think about how you can cope with these factors. Here are some ideas for strategies.

- I can't cope with the aroma of freshly baked doughnuts when I pass the baker's, so I will pass on the other side of the road.
- When the chocolate biscuits are passed round at work, I just can't resist them. But I could try offering to purchase the biscuits, and buy a type I don't find so irresistible.
- I can't live without chocolate, but I *have* discovered that just a little bit, eaten very slowly and savoured, satisfies my taste buds just as much as a whole big bar.
(Write your strategies here:)
- ....
- ....
- ....
- ....
- ....

Eating for comfort

Boredom, loneliness, misery, nervousness are all feelings that can make you want to eat. Comfort eating, as it is usually called, is a big problem. Is that your problem?

Fill out the blanks below.

Events/situations likely to make me eat when I'm not really hungry (over and above situations dealt with in previous section) are:

....

....

....

....

Here are some possible examples:

- I call up a friend to come round for the evening, but she says she's seeing another of her friends. I feel snubbed, so I eat a whole packet of biscuits.
- I'm OK all week at work, but I live alone and find Sundays very boring and lonely. I pick at food all day long.

Whatever your trigger situations – and there may be many – you need to do the following. First, replace food with something else to see you through those times. Write down here as many things as you can think of that might help (e.g., keep a diary, offer to pet-walk for neighbours, hire a video, exercise).

In trigger situations, I will:

....

....

....

....

....

Second, you need to work on the feelings that made you seek comfort in the first place. For example, in the first case, why did you feel so bad when you rang a friend and she couldn't come round? Does your self-esteem need work so that you can take the occasional 'no' without feeling a personal rejection? Are you relying on one friend too much? Why aren't you happy with your own company? Write down overleaf the reasons behind your own comfort eating problem(s).

I comfort eat because:

....

....

....

My action plan to get over it is:

....

....

....

....

The social trap

Many, many people lay the blame for over-eating firmly on their social and/or business life. They have to eat/drink more than they should, they say, because they socialise...

Why, then, do so many *slim* people manage all that – and still stay slim?

The truth is that you *can* socialise and stay slim. What slim people have is the knack of using common sense and the 'swings and roundabouts' approach to food and drink. If they eat a lot one day/evening/weekend, they tend to cut down quite naturally afterwards. This may not come very easily to some of us, but it is a great strategy to learn. The other truth is that a great deal of what you put in your mouth at any social occasion is not strictly necessary.

Here are my top strategies for socialising without putting on weight. You can think of some more.

- Home entertaining? Serve the type of low-fat high-carbohydrate food you would normally eat. Light starters and fresh fruit for dessert will keep the whole meal low in calories. Spices will make the main course more special.
- No one *has* to drink alcohol these days. Alcohol-free wines and beers or soft drinks are just as acceptable.
- Fattening set menu; no choice at all? Take small portions, refuse second helpings and avoid additions you *can* leave, such as rolls and pre-meal nibbles like crisps and nuts.

Write your socialising problems here, each one followed by your own strategy for dealing with it:

- ....

Solution: ....

....

- ....

Solution: ....

....

Never forget that you can have fun, enjoy yourself and help other people to enjoy themselves *without* eating more than you want to.

Hurting feelings

Many slimmers tell me that they over-eat because they are frightened of hurting people's feelings. A typical example is a woman who visits her mother-in-law for Sunday lunch and feels obliged to eat her way through mountains of roast potatoes, Yorkshire pudding, apple pie and double cream. There are three answers to this.

- Test the water and see if mother-in-law really will be mortally upset if you ask her for smaller portions of the fat-laden things. Nine times out of ten people aren't half as offended as you think they will be.
- Eat the lunch offered, but have only fruit for breakfast, and a big salad and a diet yoghurt for supper. Swings and roundabouts!
- Long term plan: over a period, get talking to mother-in-law about food and eating, and how you feel about your diet. Interest her in healthier eating. You could even turn the tables and have *her* not wanting to offend *you* when you come for lunch, so she prepares a meal you do find acceptable.

The deprivation factor

How often have you thought to yourself, 'I shouldn't eat that, therefore I want it all the more!'?

Wanting what we can't have is strong human motivation. So the answer is, *never* forbid yourself anything. Say, 'I *can* eat that, if I allow for it.' You plan for a little bit *often*, or a lot *occasionally*.

But, ask yourself why that food is so dear to you? If it is a high-fat, low-carbohydrate food, is it really so wonderful? Learn to think of food as fuel for your body. You give your car what it needs to run smoothly, so why not your body? Food is fuel to give you energy, and to keep you fit and healthy.

Try to work yourself through the many, many reasons you may have been eating food you didn't need and didn't even really want. You can't replace your body, so give it some thought – and plenty of quality fuel. You've *got* slim, now stay slim for the rest of your life.

FOOD CHARTS

USING THE CHARTS

On the following pages you will find my unique food charts, to help you build a low-fat, high-carbohydrate diet of good-quality food. These charts are, to my knowledge, the first charts that actually tell you how much fat, carbohydrate and protein is in every food *as a percentage of the total calories in that food*. This means that – at a glance – you can see whether what you are eating measures up to the percentage guidelines discussed in Chapter 10 i.e., up to 25 per cent of the total calories in your diet can be eaten in the form of fat and at least 60 per cent as carbohydrate calories. The remaining calories (10 to 15 per cent) can be made up by adding proteins to your diet.

All other fat charts – and food labels – have been *misleading* you, for they list the fat content as a percentage of the total *weight* of the product. Since all food contains calorie-free water, this artificially reduces the fat percentage.

Let's take some examples of what I mean. A pack of extra-lean minced beef states on the label that it contains 'only 10 per cent fat' (i.e., 10 grams of fat per 100 grams of product). You could be forgiven for thinking, then, that this is well within the 25 to 30 per cent fat guidelines we discussed earlier. In fact, of the 190 or so calories in that beef, 35 per cent of them are *fat* calories, and 65 per cent are *protein* calories. The water that the beef contains has given a false figure.

Work out this sum with Cheddar cheese, and you soon see how, if you read labels, you could easily be eating about twice as much fat as you think you are. An average packet of Cheddar cheese states 33.5 per cent fat, 26 per cent protein (or those figures in grams per 100 grams of product). That makes cheese sound only marginally high in fat, doesn't it?

In fact, the weight breakdown of the cheese is this: 37 per cent water; 33.5 per cent fat; 26 per cent protein – total calories 405. The water contains no calories, and so the calorie breakdown is: carbohydrate almost none; protein 25.5 per cent; fat 74.5 per cent. So the cheese has well over double the fat you may have thought it did.

Even 'reduced-fat' Cheddar, worked out in this way, contains 50.5 per cent fat.

Apply this to one last product: single cream, which is listed on labels and in fat charts as containing 21 per cent fat by weight. Doesn't sound too bad, does it? This equals 191 calories of fat in 100 grams of cream, but there are only 215 calories in the 100 grams of cream. So the *actual* fat content as a percentage of the total calories is a staggering 89 per cent!

My food charts tell you the *honest* truth about what you are eating. To maintain the correct fat/carbohydrate balance, then, all you need do is eat *most* of your foods from the items on the list that contain *less* than 20 per cent fat, and *plenty* of foods that contain *more* than 50 per cent carbohydrate. Eat *some* of your foods from the items that contain 20 to 30 per cent fat. And eat very *few* (or very small portions) of those that contain *over* 30 per cent fat.

The charts also list calories per portion, and they will help you to spot good sources of the vital vitamins and minerals.

Finally, I give you the grams of fat in every product listed, as a cross-reference, in case you find this helpful. If you're on an average maintenance diet of, say, 2000 calories a day, your 20 per cent fat ceiling will be 500 calories a day. This is equal to 55 grams of pure fat. So you could easily tot up your daily fat total this way and see how far off that 55 grams you are.

Just look through the lists now and see what, exactly, you have been eating!

FOOD	% FAT	% CARBOHYDRATE	% PROTEIN	CALORIES PER STATED PORTION	GRAMS OF FAT PER STATED PORTION	GOOD SOURCE OF: VITAMINS	GOOD SOURCE OF: MINERALS
Biscuits and Bars (all per biscuit or bar)							
Digestive, one large	40	52*	8	75	3.3	...	...
Digestive, chocolate, small	44	50.5*	5.5	85	4.1	...	...
Gingernut	30	65*	5	45	1.5	...	...
Harvest Crunch Bar	38	n/k	n/k	78	3.3	...	...
Rich Tea	38.5	56*	5.5	35	1.5	...	...
Shortcake (oblong)	46.5	48.5*	5	75	3.8	...	...
Breads and Crispbreads (all per 25 g [1 oz] unless otherwise stated)							
Brown	9	75	16	56	0.55	B	...
Cream cracker, one	33	58	9	40	1.5	...	...
French, white	1.2	83.3	15.5	62.5	tr	D	calcium
Malt loaf	12	74.5	13.5	62	0.82	...	iron
Oatcake, one	37	53.5	9.5	45	1.8	...	...
Pitta, white, one	4	82.5	13.5	175	0.8	...	calcium
Pitta, brown, one	7	72	21	160	1.2	...	...
Rice cake, one	7	85.5	7.5	24	0.2	...	...
Rye Granary	7.5	79.5	13	60	0.5	...	iron
Ryvita, one	11.5	77.5	11	25	0.2	...	...
Wheatgerm (e.g., Hovis)	8.5	74.5	17	57	0.55	B-group, E	iron
White	6.5	80	13.5	58	0.5	...	calcium, iron
Wholemeal	11	73	16	54	0.67	B-group	iron
Wholemeal (per slice from a large, medium-cut loaf)	11	73	16	75	0.9	B-group	iron
Wholemeal bap, one	11	73	16	120	1.5	B-group	iron

* The carbohydrate content of this product is largely, or completely, 'common sugars', or simple carbohydrate (see page 126).

† Alcohol content included in this figure.

n/k Not known.

tr Trace.

FOOD	% FAT	% CARBOHYDRATE	% PROTEIN	CALORIES PER STATED PORTION	GRAMS OF FAT PER STATED PORTION	GOOD SOURCE OF: VITAMINS	MINERALS
Breakfast Cereals (all per 25g [1 oz] unless otherwise stated)							
All Bran	18.5	59	22.5	68	1.5	B-group	iron
Bran flakes	5.5	76	12.5	80	0.5	C, D, B-group	iron
Corn flakes	4	86.5	9.5	92	0.4	B-group, D	iron
Fruit 'n Fibre	12	78	10	90	1.25	B-group, D	iron
Muesli (no added sugar)	19	71	10	82	1.7	E, B3	calcium, iron
Porridge oats, raw	22	63.5	14.5	94	2.25	...	iron
Porridge, made up with water, per 100 ml ($3^1/_2$ oz)	18	70	12	44	0.9	...	iron
Puffed wheat	3.5	79	17.5	81	0.3	...	...
Shredded wheat, one	8.5	78.5	13	80	0.75	...	...
Special K	6	75.5	18.5	97	0.6	B-group, D	iron
Weetabix, one	9	77.5	13.5	65	0.65	B3	iron
Cakes and Bakery Items (all per item or slice)							
Chocolate, rich, (small slice) 50 g (2 oz)	53	42*	5	230	13.6	...	...
Croissant, one (65 g, $2^1/_2$ oz)	54	38.5	7.5	280	16.5	...	...
Crumpet, one	3.5	83	13.5	100	0.5	...	calcium, iron
Doughnut, jam, one	41	52.5	6.5	260	12	...	...
Eclair, chocolate, one	57.5	38*	4.5	190	12	...	...
Rich fruit cake, small slice 50 g (2oz)	30	66*	4	165	5.5	A	iron
Scone, plain, one	35.5	56.5*	8	200	8	...	...
Victoria Sponge, 50 g (2oz) slice	51.5	43*	5.5	230	13.25	...	...

FOOD	% FAT	% CARBOHYDRATE	% PROTEIN	CALORIES PER STATED PORTION	GRAMS OF FAT PER STATED PORTION	GOOD SOURCE OF: VITAMINS	GOOD SOURCE OF: MINERALS
Cheese (all per 25 g [1 oz] unless otherwise stated)							
Brie or Camembert	69.5	tr	30.5	75	5.8	A, B-group, D	calcium
Cheddar	74.5	tr	25.5	101	8.3	A, B-group, D	calcium
Cheddar-style, half-fat	50.5	tr	49.5	62	3.5	A, B-group, D	calcium
Cheese spread	73	1	26	71	5.7	A, B-group, D	calcium
Cottage cheese, diet	18	tr	82	20	0.4	B2	calcium
Cottage cheese, standard	37.5	5.5	57	24	1.0	B2	calcium
Cream cheese, full fat	97	tr	3	110	12	A	...
Danish Blue	74	tr	26	89	7.3	A, B-group, D	calcium
Edam	68	tr	32	76	5.7	A, B-group, D	calcium
Mozzarella, Italian	68	3	29	62	4.75	...	calcium
Soft cheese, low-fat	57	7.5	35.5	33	2.1	...	calcium
Stilton	78	tr	22	115	10	A, B-group, D	calcium
Dressings, Sauces and Pickles (all per tbsp)							
Brown sauce	tr	95.5*	4.5	20	tr	...	...
Burger relish	tr	98	2	21	tr	...	...
French dressing	100	tr	tr	130	14.5	...	...
Mayonnaise	99	tr	1	143	15.75	...	...
Mayonnaise, reduced-calorie	89	10*	1	57	5.5	...	...
Salad cream	79	18*	3	62	5.5	...	...
Salad cream, reduced-calorie	66.5	31*	2.5	26	2	...	...
Soya sauce	6	71	23	11	tr	...	...
Sweet pickle	2	96*	2	26	tr	...	...
Tartare sauce	83	14*	3	47	4.4	...	...
Tomato ketchup	1	91*	8	20	tr	...	...
White sauce	61	27*	12	30	2	...	calcium

FOOD	% FAT	% CARBOHYDRATE	% PROTEIN	CALORIES PER STATED PORTION	GRAMS OF FAT PER STATED PORTION	GOOD SOURCE OF: VITAMINS	GOOD SOURCE OF: MINERALS
Drinks							
Alcoholic drinks							
Beer, 275 ml (1/2 pint)	tr	96.5†	3.5	90	tr	...	...
Lager, 275 ml (1/2 pint)	tr	97.5†	2.5	90	tr	...	...
Port, 25 ml (1 fl oz)	...	100†	tr	40	...	...	...
Sherry, 25 ml (1fl oz)	...	100†	tr	30	...	...	...
Spirits, all, 1 measure	...	100†	...	50	...	...	...
Stout, 275 ml (1/2 pint)	tr	100†	tr	90	tr	...	...
Wine, red, 140 ml (5 fl oz)	...	99†	1	100	...	...	...
Wine, white, medium, 140 ml (5 fl oz)	...	100†	...	100	...	...	...
Wine, white, dry 140 ml (5 fl oz)	...	100†	...	90	...	...	...
Wine, white, sweet, 140 ml (5 fl oz)	...	99†	1	140	...	...	...
Beverages							
Tea	...	tr	tr	tr	...	...	...
Coffee, one tsp	...	41	59	2.5	...	...	...
Hot chocolate, per 7 fl oz (200 ml)	19	69*	12	112	2.4	B3	calcium
Low calorie instant hot chocolate, per sachet	24	56*	20	40	1	...	...
Soft drinks							
Cola, 1 330 ml (12 fl oz) can	...	100*	...	135	...	...	...
Lemonade, one 200 ml (7 fl oz) glass	...	100*	...	50	...	...	...
Orange squash, one 200 ml (7 fl oz) glass	...	100*	...	60	...	...	...

FOOD	% FAT	% CARBOHYDRATE	% PROTEIN	CALORIES PER STATED PORTION	GRAMS OF FAT PER STATED PORTION	GOOD SOURCE OF: VITAMINS	MINERALS
Fruit Juices (all per average glass [125 ml, 4½ fl oz])							
Apple	...	97	3	50	...	...	...
Grape	...	97	3	75	...	...	...
Grapefruit	...	96	4	50	...	C	...
Mixed citrus	...	96	4	50	...	C	...
Mixed vegetable	...	85	15	25	...	C	...
Orange	...	95	5	50	...	C	...
Pineapple	...	97	3	55	...	C	...
Tomato	...	83	17	25	...	C	...
Eggs							
Size 2 (large), one egg	67	tr	33	90	6.8	A, B-group, D, E	iron, calcium
Size 3 (medium), one egg	67	tr	33	80	6	A, B-group, D, E	iron, calcium
Size 4 (small), one egg	67	tr	33	75	5.5	A, B-group, D, E	iron, calcium
Size 3 (medium), fried, drained	78	tr	22	120	10.5	A, B-group, D, E	iron, calcium
Size 3 (medium, scrambled with 7 g (¼ oz) low fat spread and 25 ml (1 fl oz) skimmed milk	64	4	32	115	9	A, B-group, D, E	iron, calcium
Fats and Oils (all per 25 g [1 oz])							
Butter	100	tr	tr	185	20.5	A, D	...
Low-fat spread	100	...	...	91	10	A, D	...
Margarine, all types, including sunflower	100	tr	tr	182	20.3	A, D	...
Oils, all kinds	100	...	tr	225	25	...	...
Very low-fat spread	100	...	...	57	6.3	A, D	...

FOOD	% FAT	% CARBOHYDRATE	% PROTEIN	CALORIES PER STATED PORTION	GRAMS OF FAT PER STATED PORTION	GOOD SOURCE OF: VITAMINS	MINERALS
Fish and Seafood (all per 100 g [3½ oz] unless otherwise stated)							
Cod, coley, haddock or monkfish fillet	8	...	92	76	0.7	B3	calcium
Deep-fried fish in batter	47	14	39	200	10.3	...	...
Fish finger, grilled, one	38	34	28	50	2	...	...
Fish, frozen, in light batter, baked or grilled, one portion, 3½ oz (100 g)	51.5	28.5	20	203	11.6	...	...
Haddock, smoked fillet	8	...	92	100	0.9	B-group	calcium
Herring fillet	71	...	29	234	18.5	B-group, D	calcium, iron
Kipper, grilled fillet	50	...	50	205	11.4	A, B-group, D	calcium, iron
Pilchards in tomato sauce	38.5	2	59.5	126	5.4	B-group, D, E	calcium
Plaice fillet	18	...	82	93	1.9	B-group	calcium
Salmon, fresh, fillet	59	...	41	197	13	A, B-group, D	...
Salmon, pink, canned	47.5	...	52.5	155	8.2	A, B-group, D, E	calcium, iron
Salmon, smoked	28.5	...	71.5	142	4.5	A, B-group, D	...
Scampi, deep-fried	50	34	16	316	17.6	...	calcium, iron
Trout, one average 225 g (8 oz)	30	...	70	200	6.75	B3	iron
Tuna in brine, drained	3	...	97	114	0.35	B-group	iron
Tuna in oil, drained	47	...	53	210	11	B-group, E	iron
Whitebait, deep fried	81	4	15	525	47.5	...	calcium, iron
Seafood							
Crabmeat	37	...	63	127	5.2	B-group	calcium
Crabmeat, canned	10	...	90	81	0.9	...	calcium, iron
Mussels, shelled	20.5	tr	79.5	87	2	...	calcium, iron
Prawns, shelled	15	...	85	107	1.8	B-group	calcium
Scallops, shelled	12	tr	88	105	1.4	...	calcium, iron
Squid	15	tr	85	82	1.4	A, B3	calcium, iron

FOOD	% FAT	% CARBOHYDRATE	% PROTEIN	CALORIES PER STATED PORTION	GRAMS OF FAT PER STATED PORTION	GOOD SOURCE OF: VITAMINS	GOOD SOURCE OF: MINERALS
Fruit (all per item, unless otherwise stated)							
Apple, dessert	tr	97	3	45	tr	...	...
Apple, cooking, per 25 g (1 oz)	tr	97	3	40	tr	...	...
Apricots, dried, per 25 g (1 oz)	tr	89.5	10.5	45	tr	A	...
Apricot, fresh	tr	93	7	10	tr	A	...
Banana, large	3.5	91	5.5	100	0.4	A, C, E	...
Banana, medium	3.5	91	5.5	80	0.3	A, C, E	...
Banana, small	3.5	91	5.5	60	0.2	A, C, E	...
Blackberries, 25 g (1 oz)	tr	83	17	7	tr	C	calcium, iron
Blackcurrants, 25 g (1 oz)	tr	88	12	7	tr	C	calcium, iron
Currants, dried, 25 g (1 oz)	tr	97	3	60	tr	...	...
Cherries, 25 g (1 oz)	tr	95	5	10	tr	...	...
Damsons, 25 g (1 oz)	tr	95	5	8	tr	...	...
Dates, each, fresh or dry	tr	96.5	3.5	15	tr	...	iron
Dates, stoned, 25 g (1 oz)	tr	96.5	3.5	62	tr	...	iron
Fig, dry	tr	93	7	53	tr	...	iron
Fig, fresh	tr	87	13	10	tr	...	iron
Gooseberries, cooking, per 25 g (1 oz)	tr	93	7	9	tr	C, E	...
Gooseberries, dessert, per 25 g (1 oz)	tr	75	25	4	tr	C, E	...
Grapefruit, half	tr	90	10	20	tr	C	...
Grapes, 25 g (1 oz)	tr	96	4	16	tr	...	...
Kiwifruit	6	86	8	25	tr	C	...
Lemon	tr	80	20	15	tr	C	...
Lime	tr	80	20	10	tr	C	...
Mango	tr	97	3	100	tr	C, A	iron
Melon, 200 g (7 oz) slice	tr	90	10	25	tr	A, C	...

FOOD	% FAT	% CARBOHYDRATE	% PROTEIN	CALORIES PER STATED PORTION	GRAMS OF FAT PER STATED PORTION	GOOD SOURCE OF: VITAMINS	MINERALS
Fruit (continued)							
Nectarine	tr	93	7	50	tr	A, B3	...
Orange	tr	92	8	50	tr	C	calcium
Peach	tr	92	8	50	tr	A	...
Pear, medium	tr	98	2	50	tr	...	...
Pineapple, one ring	tr	95	5	25	tr	C	...
Plum, one dessert	tr	94	6	20	tr	...	...
Prunes, each	tr	94	6	10	tr	A	iron
Prunes, stoned per 25 g (1 oz)	tr	94	6	40	tr	A	iron
Raisins, 25 g (1 oz)	tr	98	2	61	tr	...	...
Raspberries, 25 g (1 oz)	tr	84	16	6	tr	C	iron
Rhubarb, one large stick, 100 g (3½ oz)	tr	62.5	37.5	6	tr	C	calcium
Satsuma or tangerine	tr	91	9	20	tr	C	...
Strawberries, 25 g (1 oz)	tr	90	10	6	tr	C	iron
Sultanas, 25 g (1 oz)	tr	97	3	62	tr	...	iron
GRAINS (all per 25 g [1 oz] unless otherwise stated)							
Flour, white	3	86	11	87	0.3	...	iron, calcium
Flour, wholemeal	6	77.5	16.5	80	0.5	B3	iron
Pasta, brown (boiled weight)	8.5	72.5	18	32	0.3	...	iron
Pasta, brown, all shapes (dry weight)	7	78	15	85	0.6	...	iron
Pasta, white (boiled weight)	3	83	14	29	tr	...	iron
Pasta, white, all shapes (dry weight)	3	83	14	95	0.25	...	iron
Pearl barley (dry weight)	4	87	9	90	0.4	...	...

FOOD	% FAT	% CARBOHYDRATE	% PROTEIN	CALORIES PER STATED PORTION	GRAMS OF FAT PER STATED PORTION	GOOD SOURCE OF: VITAMINS	GOOD SOURCE OF: MINERALS
Grains (continued)							
Rice, brown (boiled weight)	7	86	7	30	0.45	B-group, E	iron
Rice, brown (dry weight)	7	85	6	90	0.7	B-group, E	iron
Rice, white (boiled weight)	2	90	8	30	tr	...	iron
Rice, white (dry weight)	2.5	90	7.5	90	0.25	...	iron
Rice salad (ready-made)	13	75	12	35	0.5	...	...
Spaghetti in tomato sauce, 213 g (7½ oz) can	10.5	77.5	12	127	1.5	...	iron
Meat and Poultry (all per 25 g [1 oz] unless otherwise stated)							
Bacon, back, trimmed, grilled	58	...	42	73	4.7	B3	...
Bacon, streaky, grilled	77	...	23	105	9	B3	...
Beef, minced	60	...	40	57	3.8	B-group	iron
Beef, minced, extra-lean	35	...	65	47	1.8	B-group	iron
Beef, roast, lean only	25	...	75	40	1.1	B-group	iron
Beef steak, lean only, grilled	32	...	68	42	1.5	B-group	...
Beefburger, one 50 g (2 oz) frozen burger, grilled	64	5	31	120	8.5	B-group	iron
Chicken, average breast with skin, 200 g (7 oz) grilled	60	...	40	225	15	B-group	iron
Chicken, average breast without skin, 200 g (7 oz) grilled	42	...	58	150	7	B-group	iron
Chicken fillet, no skin, raw	30	...	70	30	1	B-group	iron
Chicken, roast, meat only	33	...	67	37	1.3	B-group	iron
Corned beef	50	...	50	54	3	B-group, E	iron
Duck, breast fillet	46	...	54	47	2.4	B3	iron
Duck, roast, meat and skin	77	...	23	85	7.2	B3	iron

FOOD	% FAT	% CARBOHYDRATE	% PROTEIN	CALORIES PER STATED PORTION	GRAMS OF FAT PER STATED PORTION	GOOD SOURCE OF: VITAMINS	MINERALS
Meat and Poultry (continued)							
Gammon steak, grilled, lean only	27	...	73	43	1.3	B1, B3	iron
Ham, extra lean	37.5	...	62.5	30	1.25	B3	...
Kidneys, lamb's	27	...	73	22	0.67	A, B-group, E	iron
Lamb, one trimmed chop, average	50	...	50	120	6.8	B3	iron
Lamb, leg, roast, lean only	38	...	62	48	2	B3	iron
Lamb, shoulder, roast	75	...	25	80	6.5	B3	iron
Liver, lamb's	52	3	45	45	2.5	A, B-group, E	iron
Liver sausage	78	5.5	16.5	77	6.7	B-group	iron
Luncheon meat, canned pork	77.5	6.5	16	78	6.7	...	...
Pork, fillet, raw	43	...	57	37	1.75	B3	iron
Pork, roast, lean only	34	...	66	46	1.7	B3	iron
Rabbit (excluding bone)	29	...	71	31	1	B3, B12	iron
Salami	83	1	16	122	11.3	B3	...
Sausages, beef, grilled, per chipolata	59	21.5	19.5	70	4.5	B3, E	iron
Sausages, low-fat, grilled, per chipolata	43	23	34	50	2.4	B3, E	iron
Sausages, pork, grilled, per chipolata	70	13.5	16.5	75	5.8	B3, E	iron
Turkey, dark meat (no skin)	28	...	72	28	0.9	B-group	iron
Turkey, light meat (no skin)	9.5	...	90.5	26	0.3	B-group	iron
Tongue	70	...	30	53	4	B-group	iron
Veal, fillet, raw	22	...	78	27	0.6	B-group	iron
Venison, fillet	29	...	71	49	1.6	B3	iron

FOOD	% FAT	% CARBOHYDRATE	% PROTEIN	CALORIES PER STATED PORTION	GRAMS OF FAT PER STATED PORTION	GOOD SOURCE OF: VITAMINS	GOOD SOURCE OF: MINERALS
Milk and Cream (all per 25 g [1 fl oz] unless otherwise stated)							
Instant low-fat milk, dry, per tbsp	3	56	41	18	tr	D	calcium
Milk, whole	52.5	27	20.5	16	1	A, B-group	calcium
Milk, semi-skimmed	31.5	39	29.5	11.5	0.4	B-group	calcium
Milk, skimmed	2	57	41	8	tr	B-group	calcium
Soya milk	53.5	10	36.5	8	0.5	D	calcium
Aerosol cream	87	10	3	16	1.5	...	calcium
Double cream	97	1.5	1.5	112	12	D	calcium
Single cream	90	5.5	4.5	53	5.3	D	calcium
Sour cream	88	7	5	51	5	D	calcium
Nuts and Crisps (all per 25 g [1oz], shelled weight)							
Almonds	85	3	12	141	13.3	E	calcium
Brazils	89.5	2.5	8	155	15.3	E	...
Chestnuts	14	81	5	42	0.67	...	...
Hazelnuts	85	7	8	95	9	E	...
Peanuts, fresh or dry-roasted	77.5	5.5	17	142	12. 2	E, B3	...
Walnuts	89	3	8	131	9	...	...
Crisps, standard	60.5	34.5	5	133	9	...	...
Lower-fat crisps	56	36.5	7.5	105	6.5	...	...
Pastry and Pizza							
Cornish pasty, one small, 130 g ($4^{1}/_{2}$ oz)	55.5	35	9.5	430	26.5	...	...
Filo, 25 g (1 oz)	9.5	78	12.5	67	0.7	...	...
Flaky, 25 g (1 oz)	64.5	31.5	4	106	7.6	...	...

FOOD	% FAT	% CARBOHYDRATE	% PROTEIN	CALORIES PER STATED PORTION	GRAMS OF FAT PER STATED PORTION	GOOD SOURCE OF: VITAMINS	MINERALS
Pastry and Pizza (continued)							
Jam tart, one	35	61*	4	150	5.8	...	...
Mince pie, one	43	53*	4	200	9.5	...	...
Pork pie, one individual, 140 g (5 oz)	64.5	25	10.5	530	37.8	B3	iron
Quiche, one slice, 100 g (3½ oz)	65	20	15	390	28	A	calcium, iron
Sausage roll, one large	68	26	6	270	20.5	...	...
Shortcrust, 25 g (1 oz)	55	40	5	113	7	...	...
Steak and kidney, one individual, 130 g (4½ oz)	59	30	11	480	31.5	A, B12	iron

Puddings and Desserts

FOOD	% FAT	% CARBOHYDRATE	% PROTEIN	CALORIES PER STATED PORTION	GRAMS OF FAT PER STATED PORTION	VITAMINS	MINERALS
Black Forest gateau, per 100 g (3½ oz) portion	53	42*	5	310	18.2	...	...
Cheesecake, per 50 g (2 oz) portion	75	21*	4	210	17.5	A	calcium
Custard, ready-made, 100 ml (3½ oz)	34	53*	13	120	4.5	...	calcium
Fruit pie, per 100 g (3½ oz) portion	38	57.5*	4.5	180	7.6	...	...
Ice cream, vanilla, per 50 g (2 oz) portion	35.5	55.5*	9	83	3.3	...	calcium
Trifle, per 100 g (3½ oz) portion	34	57*	9	160	6.1	A	calcium

FOOD	% FAT	% CARBOHYDRATE	% PROTEIN	CALORIES PER STATED PORTION	GRAMS OF FAT PER STATED PORTION	GOOD SOURCE OF: VITAMINS	GOOD SOURCE OF: MINERALS
Pulses, Beans, Peas and Lentils (all per 25 g [1 oz])							
Baked beans in tomato sauce	6	61	33	16	0.1	E	iron, calcium
Butter beans, canned or boiled	2.5	67.5	30	23	tr	E	iron
Chick peas, canned or boiled	18	60	22	40	0.8	E	iron
Haricot beans, canned or boiled	5	67	28	23	0.1	E	iron
Kidney beans, canned or boiled	4.5	59.5	36	25	0.1	...	iron
Lentils, dry weight	3	65.5	31.5	76	0.25	...	iron
Lentils, boiled	4.5	64.5	31	25	0.1	...	iron
Split peas, boiled	2.5	69.5	28	30	tr	...	iron
Soups (all per 300 g [11 oz] serving)							
Cream of chicken	59	29	12	175	11.5	...	...
Cream of tomato	45	46	9	173	8.7	...	...
Lentil	2.5	72.5	25	115	0.3	...	iron
Minestrone	29.5	55	15.5	90	2.9	...	...
Vegetable	14.5	72.5	13	110	1.8	...	...
Spreads (all per 25 g [1 oz] unless otherwise stated)							
Jam	...	99*	1	65	...	...	...
Liver pâté	67.5	1.5	31	80	6	A, B12	iron
Marmalade	...	100*	tr	65	...	...	...

FOOD	% FAT	% CARBOHYDRATE	% PROTEIN	CALORIES PER STATED PORTION	GRAMS OF FAT PER STATED PORTION	GOOD SOURCE OF: VITAMINS	MINERALS
Spreads (continued)							
Marmite, per tsp	3.5	4	92.5	9	tr	B-group	...
Peanut butter	77.5	8	14.5	156	13.4	E, B3	...
Taramasalata	94	3.5	2.5	110	11.5	...	...
Sugars and Confectionery (all per 25 g [1 oz] unless otherwise stated)							
Chocolate, milk or plain	51.5	42*	6.5	132	7.5	...	...
Honey	...	99.5*	0.5	72	...	...	...
Sugar	...	100*	...	98	...	...	...
Sugar, per tsp	...	100*	...	20	...	...	...
Sweets, boiled	...	100*	...	82	...	...	...
Syrup	...	100*	...	75	...	...	...
Toffee	36	62*	2	107	4.3	...	...
Vegetables (all per 25 g [1 oz] unless otherwise stated)							
Artichoke, globe, one whole (edible parts)	1	70	29	15	tr	...	...
Artichoke, Jerusalem	tr	64.5	35.5	4.5	tr	...	...
Asparagus, one spear, 50 g (2 oz)	tr	24	75.5	4.5	tr	E, C	iron
Aubergine	tr	80	20	3.5	tr	...	...
Avocado, half medium, 65g ($2^1/_2$ oz)	89	3	8	145	14.4	E, C	iron
Beans, broad	10.5	55.5	34	12	0.1	A, C, B3	iron
Beans, French	tr	59	41	10	tr	A	...
Beans, runner	7	53	40	5	tr	A	...
Beansprouts	tr	29	71	7	tr	...	...

FOOD	% FAT	% CARBOHYDRATE	% PROTEIN	CALORIES PER STATED PORTION	GRAMS OF FAT PER STATED PORTION	GOOD SOURCE OF: VITAMINS	MINERALS
Vegetables (continued)							
Beetroot	tr	84	16	11	tr	...	...
Broccoli	tr	31	69	4.5	tr	A, C, E	iron, calcium
Brussels sprouts	tr	36	62	4.5	tr	A, C, E	...
Cabbage, dark	tr	50	50	6	tr	A, C, E	iron
Cabbage, red	tr	66	34	5	tr	C	calcium
Cabbage, white	tr	65	35	5	tr	C	...
Carrots	tr	88	12	6	tr	A, E	calcium
Cauliflower	tr	42	58	3	tr	C	...
Celery	tr	61	39	2	tr	...	...
Chicory	tr	62	38	2	tr	...	...
Chinese leaves	tr	50	50	3	tr	C, A	iron
Corn on the cob, one	17	70	13	80	1.5	A	...
Courgettes	3.5	67.5	29	5	0.1	A, C	iron
Cucumber	9	67	24	2	tr	...	...
Leek	tr	72	28	8	tr	C, E	iron, calcium
Lettuce	30	37.5	32.5	3	0.1	...	...
Marrow	tr	87	13	4	tr	...	...
Mushrooms	41.5	...	55	3	0.1	...	...
Mustard and cress, whole box	tr	34	64	5	tr	A	...
Onion	tr	85	15	6	tr	C	...
Onion, spring, one	tr	91	9	3	tr	...	...
Parsnip	tr	86.5	13.5	12	tr	E	...
Peas, shelled, fresh or frozen	7	55	38	13	0.1	C	iron
Pepper, green	22.5	53.5	24	4	0.1	A, C, E	...
Pepper, other colours	11	77	12	8	0.1	A, C, E	...
Potatoes:							
Baked, average, 225 g (8 oz)	1	89.5	9.5	190	0.2	C	iron
Boiled	1	92	7	20	tr	C	...

FOOD	% FAT	% CARBOHYDRATE	% PROTEIN	CALORIES PER STATED PORTION	GRAMS OF FAT PER STATED PORTION	GOOD SOURCE OF: VITAMINS	MINERALS
Vegetables (continued)							
Potatoes *(continued)*:							
Chips, average cut, 25 g (1 oz)	41.5	55	3.5	65	3	...	...
Chips, oven	32	62.5	5.5	49	1.75	...	...
Instant mashed (made up)	9.5	79	11.5	16	0.2	C	...
Mashed	38	57	5	30	1.25	C	...
Roast, one chunk, 50 g (2 oz)	27.5	65	7.5	80	2.4	C	iron
Radish	tr	70	30	4	tr	C	iron
Spinach	14.5	17.5	68	7	0.1	A, C, E	calcium, iron
Swede	tr	77	13	5	tr	C	...
Sweet potato	6.5	88.5	5	21	0.15	A, C, E	...
Sweetcorn kernels	15	69.5	15.5	30	0.5	A	...
Tomato, one average, 50 g (2 oz)	tr	75	25	7	tr	A, C, E	...
Tomatoes, canned	1	62.5	36.5	3	tr	A, C, E	iron
Turnip	22	62	16	4	0.1	C	calcium, iron
Watercress	tr	17	83	3	tr	A, C	calcium, iron
Vegetarian Products							
Nut loaf, 100 g (3½ oz)	41	41	18	210	9.5	...	...
Quorn, 25 g (1 oz)	34	8	58	21	0.8	n/k	n/k
Sosmix, made up, 100 g (3½ oz)	59	24	17	170	11.2	...	calcium, iron
Tofu, 25 g (1 oz)	53	3	44	17	1	...	calcium, iron
TVP mince, reconstituted weight, 25 g (1 oz)	2.5	39	58.5	17	tr	...	calcium, iron
Vegeburger, 50 g (2 oz) burger	45	22.5	32.5	81	4	...	calcium, iron

FOOD	% FAT	% CARBOHYDRATE	% PROTEIN	CALORIES PER STATED PORTION	GRAMS OF FAT PER STATED PORTION	GOOD SOURCE OF: VITAMINS	MINERALS
Yoghurt and Fromage Frais (all per 25 g [1 oz] unless otherwise stated)							
Fromage frais, diet fruit, 100 g ($3^1/_2$ oz)	2	39.5	58.5	43	0.1	...	calcium
Fromage frais, fruit	27	48*	25	28	0.85	...	calcium
Fromage frais, natural (8 % fat)	64	9	27	28	2	...	calcium
Fromage frais, natural, very-low-fat	4	22	74	12	tr	...	calcium
Yoghurt, diet fruit, 125 g ($4^1/_2$ oz)	2	54	44	51	0.1	...	calcium
Yoghurt, fruit	9.5	70.5*	20	24	0.25	...	calcium
Yoghurt, natural, low-fat	13.5	48	38.5	13	0.25	...	calcium
Yoghurt, natural, whole-milk	52	25	23	17	1	...	calcium
Yoghurt, strained Greek	61	n/k	n/k	33	2.25	...	calcium

* The carbohydrate content of this product is largely, or completely, 'common sugars', or simple carbohydrate (see page 126).
† Alcohol content included in this figure.
n/k Not known.
tr Trace.

Index of Recipes

Beef
Chilli Con Carne 69
Chilli Peppers 68
Savoury Minced Beef 68
Speedy Bolognese Sauce 58

Caribbean Chicken 67
Cheesy Chicken and Pasta 60
Cheesy Vegetable Bake 62
Chicken
Caribbean Chicken 67
Cheesy Chicken and Pasta 60
Chicken and Broccoli in Yellow Bean Sauce 66
Chilli Chicken with Aromatic Rice 66
Chicken Brochettes 67
Lemon Chicken Stir-fry 66
Nutty Chicken with Beansprouts 68
Tangy Grilled Chicken 67
Thai Chicken 67
Chicken and Broccoli in Yellow Bean Sauce 66
Chicken Brochettes 67
Chilli Chicken with Aromatic Rice 66
Chilli Con Carne 69
Chilli Peppers 68
Chow Mein 59
Cod Creole 64
Curry Sauce 58

Eggs
Ratatouille with Egg 63

Fish
Cod Creole 64
Fish Moussaka 63
Haddock and Spinach Layer 65
Prawn and Mushroom Risotto 59
Rice Salad with Tuna 60
Sweet and Sour Stir-fry 65
Tandoori Fish Kebabs 64
Tuna and Broccoli Bake 64
Tuna Fish Cakes 64
Fish Moussaka 63

Haddock and Spinach Layer 65

Lamb
Lamb Burgers 69
Lamb Burgers 69
Lemon Chicken Stir-fry 66

Macaroni and Chick Peas 61
Meat-free Bolognese sauce 58
Mushroom and Tomato Sauce 57
Mushroom Risotto, and Prawn 59
Mushroom Risotto, and Tofu 59
Mushroom Risotto, and Tuna 59

Nut Pilaff 60
Nutty Chicken with Beansprouts 68

Pasta
Cheesy Chicken and Pasta 60
Chow Mein 59
Cod Creole 64
Macaroni and Chick Peas 61
Red Pepper Pasta 61
Tomato and Ham Tagliatelle 59
Pea Soup 58
Pork
Pork and Pineapple Sir-fry 69
Potato and Ham Stir-fry 62
Potato Soup 58
Prawn and Mushroom Risotto 59
Pulses
Macaroni and Chick Peas 61
Savoury Lentil Crumble 62
Speedy Bolognese Sauce 58

Ratatouille with Egg 63
Red Pepper Pasta 61
Rice
Chilli Chicken with Aromatic Rice 66
Nut Pilaff 60
Prawn and Mushroom Risotto 59
Rice Salad with Tuna 60
Vegetable Rice 60
Rice Salad with Tuna 60
Risotto, Prawn and Mushroom 59

Sauces
Curry Sauce 58
Speedy Bolognese Sauce 58
Tomato Sauce 57
Savoury Lentil Crumble 62
Savoury Minced Beef 68
Soups
Pea Soup 58
Potato Soup 58
Speedy Bolognese Sauce 58
Sweet and Sour Stir-fry 65

Tagliatelle, Tomato and Ham 59
Tandoori Fish Kebabs 64
Tangy Grilled Chicken 67
Thai Chicken 67
Tofu, and Mushroom Risotto 59
Tomato and Ham Tagliatelle 59
Tomato Sauce 57
with mushrooms 57
Tuna and Broccoli Bake 64
Tuna, and Mushroom Risotto 59
Tuna Fish Cakes 64

Vegetarian
Cheesy Vegetable Bake 62
Chilli Peppers (Variation) 68
Chow Mein 59
Macaroni and Chick Peas 61
Nut Pilaff 60
Potato Stir-fry, and red kidney beans 62
Ratatouille with Egg 63
Red Pepper Pasta (Variation) 61
Savoury Lentil Crumble 62
Savoury Minced Beef (Variation) 68
Vegetarian chilli 69
Vegetable Curry 63
Vegetable Rice 60